I MARRIED A

*N*utritionist

THINGS I'VE LEARNED THAT EVERY GUY SHOULD KNOW

Copyright © 2012 Karen Roth Nutrition, Inc.

Printed in the United States of America

1st printing – 2012

ISBN: 978-0-9854264-0-8

Cover and interior book design by: James Arneson of Jaad Book Design

Cover photo by: Steven Bridges

Edited by: Robin Quinn

Contact

- Email: IMarriedaNutritionist@gmail.com
- Website/Book: IMarriedaNutritionist.com
- Website/Karen: KarenRothNutrition.com
- Facebook Page: Facebook.com/IMarriedaNutritionistBook
- Twitter/Karen: @KarenRothMSNC
- Twitter/Steve: @HealthySpouse
- YouTube: YouTube.com/NutritionalChoice

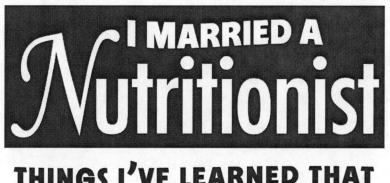

I MARRIED A Nutritionist

THINGS I'VE LEARNED THAT EVERY GUY SHOULD KNOW

STEVE ROTH

KAREN ROTH

MS, CNC

Holistic Nutritionist

"The way some guys treat their body, you'd think they were renting."
~ Robert Brault

Disclaimer

The material in this book is for informational purposes only and is not intended for the treatment or diagnosis of individual disease or other health conditions. Please visit a qualified medical or other health professional for specific diagnosis and treatment of any ailments mentioned or discussed in this book.

This book is not meant to serve as medical advice and should not be interpreted to replace the necessity for diagnosis and direct management by a qualified healthcare provider.

Dedication

We dedicate this book to all the hard-working nutritionists, naturopaths, and holistic practitioners who are often challenged by the medical establishment, big pharma, and special-interest-driven government regulations in their effort to educate, bring change, open closed minds, and truly heal.

We dedicate this book to the thousands of healthy food manufacturers who fight tooth and nail to develop, promote, and distribute products that contain safe and natural ingredients that don't harm people and other living things.

We dedicate this book to all the farmers who bring us locally grown, non-GMO organic food as well as clean, hormone-free meat and dairy products. It's not only better for us, it tastes better!

We dedicate this book to grocery retailers who understand that providing their customers with healthy products is not just good for business, it also keeps their customer base healthy so they can live longer and buy more products over the long haul.

Finally, we dedicate this book to you, our readers, who are interested in learning how to improve your health through smarter, informed choices.

Cheers,

Steve & Karen

TABLE OF CONTENTS

INTRODUCTION STUFF

YOU HAVE TO BEGIN SOMEWHERE

Steve: Okay, guys. I know what you're thinking. Marry a nutritionist and get 24/7 free advice on staying healthy. Well, that's true. Sometimes it's advice I ask for, such as when I forget the difference between organic chicken versus cage-free and hormone-free, or the difference between good and bad cholesterol. Other times the advice I receive may be unsolicited in the form of a raised eyebrow or a glare that says, "I can't believe you're eating that." But, overall, being married to a nutritionist is a good thing.

Karen: In your case ... definitely.

Steve: Okay, I can see already where this book is headed. Guys ... meet Karen, my wife and nutritionist.

Karen: Hello everyone.

Steve: Okay, that's enough. Now, as I was saying ...

Karen: Excuse me?

Steve: C'mon. I gotta keep this train moving. You know guys ...

Karen: You mean their limited attention span?

Steve: No. The fact that guys are busy and we have a lot of important things to share. Did you just roll your eyes?

Karen: No, just something in my eye.

Steve: She rolled her eyes. Now, as I was saying ... the things I've learned by being married to a nutritionist will no doubt add years to my life and help me avoid going on medications to lower my cholesterol and/or blood pressure, something many of my male friends are on. And speaking of Statins and Beta

Blockers, my nutritionist informed me that when guys are taking these pharmaceuticals, they also need to be taking something called coenzyme Q-10 … or Co-Q10 for short. Why? Because Statins and Beta Blockers reduce this vital nutrient in your body. How about that? Our book's first big piece of advice!

Karen: Okay, that was good.

Steve: Thank you.

Karen: But don't forget to mention that without Co-Q10, we humans would not have enough energy to fuel the physiological reactions we need to survive. Think of Co-Q10 as the spark plug that generates energy in our body.

Steve: That's exactly what I was going to say … the spark plug thing.

Karen: Of course you were.

Steve: So, as I was saying … if Co-Q10 is so important, why aren't more guys on Statins taking it? The reality is, most guys don't read labels and very few doctors take the time to point it out. Just like doctors forgetting to mention that side effects of Statins may include Erectile Dysfunction and your penis getting smaller.

Karen: I'm glad you're not on Statins.

Steve: Tell me about it. Now, my goal for writing this book with Karen is simple. I want to share with you guys out there some important things I've learned from my live-in nutritionist about food and nutrition which may not only improve your health, but make you live longer.

Karen: And healthier.

Steve: Right. I'm glad you've decided to take this ride because we have some things in our arsenal that may make this one of the most important books you've ever read. And what you learn from this book, we hope you'll share with your buddies so they, too, may live long lives and you'll be able to go on more guy adventures together in your old age. Never underestimate how much fun, and trouble, grey-haired guys can get into together … IF they stay healthy. Anything to add?

Karen: I think we're good. After all, like you said, these guys are busy.

Steve: Indeed they are. Rock n' roll. Let's get started …

Karen: Chapter One.

Steve: Aw, c'mon. I wanted to introduce the first chapter.

Karen: Too late. It's out in the world.

Steve: Chapter One. THE BIG STUFF. Ha! You didn't say the whole title!

Karen: Didn't have to. Everyone knows you start with what's most important.

Steve: Last word thing, huh?

Karen: Yup.

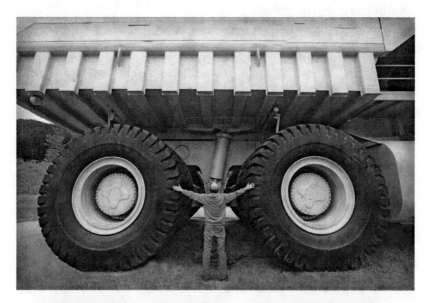

THE BIG STUFF
CHAPTER 1

*"Enjoy the little things, for one day you may look back and realize they were the big things." ~ **Robert Brault***

"I think Robert Brault is right. High school gym class wasn't fair, especially when you compared yourself with the biggest kid in the shower room."
~ Steve Roth

Sugar and Those Silly Substitutes

Steve: Okay, let's start right out of the gate with a bunker-buster, something so startling it may in fact cause you to put down your cola. The average person consumes 158 pounds of sugar per year. That's *3 pounds* of sugar per week. What? You gotta be kidding? I wish I were. Sugar is hidden in many of the foods we eat, such as luncheon meat, soup, yogurt, bread, cereal, peanut butter, frozen entrees, crackers, even in a lot of toothpaste which we use to get the sugar *off* our teeth. Go figure. Roughly 80% of the sugar we ingest comes from hidden sources.

Karen: Makes you want to start reading labels, doesn't it?

Steve: I don't know about you guys, but for me, food labels can be confusing. With that in mind, here's what I learned from Karen about reading food labels. When it comes to sugar, for every 4 grams of sugar listed on a food label, you are consuming 1 teaspoon of sugar and 15 calories. So when you take a look at that low-fat yogurt you're eating, and it says 24 grams of sugar per serving, guess what? You're downing 6 teaspoons of sugar per "serving," no matter how healthy they say it is on the packaging. Just to recap … 4 grams = 1 teaspoon = 15 calories. Or remember it this way: 4 … 1 … 15 … Hike!

Karen: You're such a guy.

Steve: I'll take that as a compliment, thank you. Now, guys, dumping all that sugar into your cake hole does a number on your body. And through cause and effect, your body may retaliate with water retention, headaches, mental sluggishness, depression, dizziness, irritability, weight gain, and insomnia. Sounds like a drug commercial, doesn't it? Side effects may include blah, blah, blah.

Karen: Unlike the pharmaceutical companies which are obligated by law to tell you their product's side effects, the FDA and the food manufacturers aren't so eager to discuss what these hidden sugars can do to you.

Steve: Those bastards!

Karen: A little over the top, but I like your enthusiasm.

Steve: Thank you. Now, if you're like me, you're probably wondering how they get that much sugar in food. Well, one of the biggest ways is something called high fructose corn syrup, which is 20-times sweeter than white table sugar. I'm sure you've been hearing a lot about it in the news as a big contributing factor in making Americans super-sized.

Karen: By just saying "NO" to high fructose corn syrup, you can instantly improve your overall health.

Steve: Big tip there, right from the nutritionist. And guess what else? When you dump all that sugar into your body, you're suppressing your immune system for up to 6 hours. And when your shield is down, you're much more likely to get attacked by all the things out there that like to take us down, like germs, colds, and infections. Excess sugar in your system also turns to fat, increases your triglycerides and cholesterol, and all that action helps promote Heart Disease. Gee, you think there could be a correlation between everyone having heart attacks and hidden sugar in foods? We'll let you make that conclusion.

Karen: Hidden sugars go by a lot of names. You should become familiar with this list:

▶ Any ingredient coupled with the word "syrup" (corn syrup, maple syrup, malt syrup, corn syrup solids, etc.)

▶ Any ingredient paired with the word "sugar" (beet sugar, brown sugar, cane sugar, corn sugar, date sugar, maple sugar, confectioner's sugar, granulated sugar, invert sugar, turbinado sugar, table sugar, raw sugar, corn starch sugar)

▶ High fructose corn syrup

▶ Molasses

▶ Any ingredient ending in "ose" (sucrose, glucose, maltose, fructose, dextrose)

▶ Cane juice concentrate

▶ Honey

▶ Sweet sorghum

- Corn sweeteners
- Dextrin
- Evaporated cane juice
- Fruit juice concentrate
- Maltodextrin

Steve: With so many sugar ingredients disguising themselves under all these names, it's no wonder everyone is confused. Okay, now we're going to roll up our sleeves and dive into the truth about artificial sweeteners.

Karen: If this were an audio book, you would now hear horror music.

Steve: I like that. Well put.

Karen: Artificial Sweeteners, you know the names ... Splenda, NutraSweet, Equal, Sweet-N-Low, and Sugar Twin ... and two you may never have heard about...Sunett or Sweet One and Neotame.

Steve: But wait! Isn't Splenda made from sugar and therefore okay?

Karen: Splenda made from sugar? Hardly. That's just effective marketing.

Steve: Let's start off by taking a closer look. Believe it or not, Splenda is 600-times sweeter than sugar. Because you need so little, and the standard sugar packet is so big, it's mixed with, huh ... *sugar* to fill up the packet. It's 99% sugar and 1% sucralose.

Karen: Now here's where I have problems with the product. A packet of Splenda claims to be sugar-free and calorie-free when in fact each packet has 4 calories and .4 grams of sugar.

Steve: How's that possible?

Karen: The law allows food makers to claim "calorie-free" if there's less than 5 calories per serving. In this case, each packet is a serving and they're allowed to claim "sugar-free" if it contains a half-gram or less of sugar per serving.

Steve: And this can have a consequence, especially if you're Diabetic and restricting sugar intake.

Karen: But that's the least of your worries. You should know that sucralose, or Splenda, is in the category of chemicals called "organochlorines," which also include DDT, mustard gas, and chloroform. I think we'll leave it at that.

Steve: Next up to bat ... aspartame, otherwise known as NutraSweet and Equal. These two products have been on the market for quite some time and both are 200-times sweeter than sugar. Not quite the powerhouse sweetening concentrate of Splenda but something that still packs a punch.

Karen: Here's something many people don't realize about aspartame. When it's absorbed into the bloodstream, it's broken down into methanol or wood alcohol. The methanol is then metabolized into formaldehyde.

Steve: The EPA says you're safe with 7.8 milligrams of methanol per day. The only problem is, one diet soda delivers almost 16 milligrams of methanol so right there you've maxed out your maximum two times over. So remember this, if you want to comply with the EPA's safety levels, only drink the top half of that can of diet soda. The other half? Well, if it's a cola, you can always pour it on your car battery to eat away that foamy white corrosion that's been building up.

Karen: There have been over seven thousand documented consumer complaints filed with the FDA about these aspartame products, and when you read some of the complaints below, you'll begin to see how these products don't sit well with your body.

- Headaches and migraines
- Dizziness and problems with balance
- Memory loss
- Fatigue
- Breathing difficulties
- Joint and bone pain
- Eye irritation
- Muscle tremors
- Wheezing
- Constipation
- Sinus problems
- Dilated eyes
- Temporary blindness
- Hallucinations
- A host of other problems

Steve: Let's talk about something made by NutraSweet called Neotame, which is based on the aspartame formula. Get this, Neotame is 13,000-times sweeter than table sugar and about 30-times sweeter than aspartame. Neotame is like aspartame on steroids!

Karen: Neotame is essentially aspartame plus 3,3-dimethylbutyl, which is a highly flammable irritant that carries risk statements for handling including irritating to skin, eyes, and respiratory system.

Steve: Oh, yeah. Now there's a sweetener I want in my food.

Karen: As Dr. Joseph Mercola pointed out in his recent blog, "Is This More-Dangerous-than-Aspartame Sweetener Hiding in Your Food?" … Neotame, under the brand name Sweetos, is used in India as a substitute for molasses in cattle feed. According to a press release, cattle consume more feed when it's mixed with Sweetos. So there goes that long-held belief that artificial sweeteners are useful in weight loss. Like aspartame, Neotame has the potential to cause weight gain because it can raise your insulin and leptin levels, two hormones responsible for Obesity, Diabetes, and many other chronic diseases.

Steve: Neotame is more stable at high temperatures than aspartame, so it's approved for use in a wider array of food products, including baked goods.

Karen: Remember, one way to avoid artificial sweeteners such as Neotame is to purchase foods bearing the USDA 100% Organic label.

Steve: Batting in the third position is Sweet 'n Low and Sugar Twin. Weighing in at 300-times sweeter than sugar is that age-old artificial sweetener our parents grew to love, saccharin. Numerous studies have shown that saccharin boosts insulin levels, creates sugar cravings, and even causes withdrawal symptoms. Enough said.

Karen: It's now common knowledge that artificial sweeteners don't help with weight loss. They only stimulate the need for more sugar so we eat more foods, get fat, need to diet, and use more ... artificial sweeteners.

Steve: Okay, let's get back to that last one you mentioned.

Karen: Acesculfame potassium?

Steve: That's the one.

Karen: You'll see acesculfame potassium abbreviated as Ace-K and it's often coupled with aspartame and/or sucralose. Although it's generally used as an ingredient in many products like gums, mints, and bottled beverages, it can be found under the brand name Sweet One in consumer packets. Ace-K may have residues of a known Cancer-causing chemical that is part of the manufacturing process.

Steve: As the Church Lady says, "Isn't that special." Now that we've totally driven you into a deep, dark depression, here's a lifeline. You *do* have options when it comes to sweeteners. In fact, some of the options are actually good for you, rats, mice, and other living things.

Karen: First up to bat for "Team Healthy" is stevia, which is 200 to 300 times sweeter than sugar. It's a very sweet herb from South America that's available in most supermarkets in powder and liquid form. This herb has been used for hundreds of years, is sugar-free, calorie-free, and is zero on the Glycemic Index. Stevia can be used to sweeten beverages and is safe for Diabetics. The spice-size container that Steve uses for his coffee and cocoa comes with a tiny little scoop, smaller than a pencil eraser.

Steve: One scoop sweetens a whole cup. It does change the flavor of coffee a tiny bit but after you use it for a while you probably won't even notice. And with 1,120 servings per spice-size bottle, that little container lasts a very long time.

Karen: Xylitol is another alternative sweetener. It was discovered in 1891, is derived from plant sources, and has 50% fewer calories than sugar.

Steve: Looks and tastes just like sugar.

Karen: Xylitol is low-calorie, only 7 on the Glycemic Index, and is great for baking. It measures teaspoon for teaspoon to sugar and is safe for Diabetics. Now here's where xylitol takes a right turn from sugar; it actually "reduces" tooth decay. Don't use too much, though. Xylitol may have a laxative effect in some people when consumed in excess, such as 3 or more teaspoons at one time.

Steve: So use xylitol responsibly or you may find yourself doing an end run at your next Super Bowl party.

Karen: What is it with guys and toilet humor?

Steve: An art form … or fart form, I can't remember.

Karen: One more note on xylitol. Make sure your pets don't eat it or products made from xylitol. What's good for humans can be really bad for pets.

Okay, the final natural sweetener is erythritol. A natural sweetener manufactured from corn starch, erythritol is 70% as sweet as sugar, is calorie-free and sugar-free. It's zero on the Glycemic Index and has no laxative effect. Erythritol is great for sweetening beverages and baked goods.

Steve: Bottom line, guys. When you want to sweeten things, first choose *stevia*, *xylitol*, and *erythritol*. If they're not available, choose *raw sugar*. If that's not available, chose *regular sugar*. If that's not available, man up and go without. *Avoid artificial sweeteners like the plague.*

Soy Is No Joy

Steve: Okay, before we dig into the soy situation, let's talk a little bit about hormones. And I'm now glancing over at Karen because that's one of her areas of expertise.

Karen: The important hormone for guys is testosterone.

Steve: See what I mean, guys? Is she an expert or what?

Karen: As I was saying …

Steve: Before you were rudely interrupted …

Karen: Yes. The important hormone for men is testosterone.

Steve: And we guys know that name because it's often associated with man caves, X-Games, grunting like Tim Allen, and working out at the gym.

Karen: In the right amount, testosterone is vital to good health in men.

Steve: Absolutely. It keeps our bodies looking like guys, you know, with hair in all the right places.

Karen: And wrong places.

Steve: Not our fault. Remember, we were once cave men.

Karen: Once?

Steve: Testosterone also gives us guys muscle tone that generally keeps us looking, you know, un-woman like. It is also the most important of the male sex hormones.

Karen: The same way estrogen is the key hormone for women.

Steve: And let me just say on behalf of all the guys out there, we appreciate estrogen in women. It makes their chests bigger than ours, skin looking ever so smooth, and a host of other physical and emotional things that keep women from being, you know, man like.

Karen: Many men are surprised to learn that their bodies produce and circulate small amounts of estrogen. But that's a good thing for men because it helps provide hormonal balance and healthy body function.

Steve: Which brings us back around to the topic of soy. In many of its forms, soy contains something called phytoestrogens, which is a long fancy name for plant estrogens.

Karen: And when men and women eat too much soy it boosts their estrogen levels and lowers testosterone.

Steve: And while we mentioned that it is okay for guys to have "some" estrogen in their systems, having a lot of it dumped into our bodies isn't necessarily a good thing. And lowering our testosterone definitely is not good.

Karen: Absolutely. Studies have suggested that excessive estrogen in men's systems can cause a host of problems including low sperm count and even what guys refer to as "man boobs."

Steve: You said boobs.

Karen: Okay, "man breasts."

Steve: I like boobs better.

Karen: Other research questions those studies. However, as reported on the news website *Science Daily,* a prospective population-based study found that higher estrogen levels in older men may be associated with an increased risk of Dementia.

Steve: Which could mean that if you have man boobs, you might just forget they're there.

Karen: Feeding children too much soy can also be a problem as their bodies develop. When young boys consume soy foods and are exposed to high levels of phytoestrogens, it can delay their sexual development. Young girls will experience premature sexual development.

Steve: What was it that you told me about monks and tofu?

Karen: According to The Weston A. Price Organization, tofu is consumed by Buddhist monks to reduce libido.

Steve: Makes sense. Can't be pitching a tent under those robes. It looks like you're stealing candle sticks.

Karen: And Japanese housewives frequently feed tofu to their husbands when they want to reduce their virility.

Steve: Ah, the old slip the husband some tofu so he doesn't in turn slip her the old baloney. I bet seeing tofu on your dinner plate speaks louder than "I have a headache."

Karen: You never know.

Steve: But there are some good kinds of soy, right?

Karen: Yes. Soy that's been fermented such as miso, tempeh, soy sauce and natto. Unfortunately, tofu and the mountains of soy food additives Americans consume daily, by choice or ignorance, is unfermented.

Steve: What do you mean by ignorance?

Karen: Well, if you look at the labels of the most common foods, you will see soy in almost everything. Soy flour in bread products, soy oil in salad dressings and marinades, soy protein isolate in protein bars and shakes, soy lecithin in candy, ice cream, butter substitutes, and much more. And the soy used in many of the products you buy in the grocery store is often genetically modified and heavily processed.

Steve: Bottom line, guys ... Organic Fermented Soy, like miso or tempeh, good. Processed Soy, such as soy milk and soy burgers bad. And people who consume too much soy are creating excessive estrogen in the body and for men, as well as women, that's not a good thing.

Karen: Well, I think that just about covers it.

Steve: Actually, there's just one more thing. Guys, if your wife is suddenly force-feeding you tofu, she's either clueless about the affects, or ready for a vacation from Hector Erector the Cervix Inspector.

The Big O - Organic

Steve: Making sense of what "organic" means drives consumers out of their minds.

Karen: Don't you think that's a little over the top? Out of their minds?

Steve: Okay, then … how about wacko?

Karen: Like you sometimes.

Steve: Absolutely. I wear my wacko badge proudly.

Karen: Yes, you do.

Steve: In today's economy, many people are changing their buying habits at the grocery store to save money. I know we are.

Karen: And, at the same time, people are looking to reduce their exposure to harmful pesticides found in the foods they eat. By understanding which fruits and vegetables contain the most and least amount of Cancer-causing chemicals, you can prioritize what foods to buy organic.

Steve: Today the Environmental Protection Agency considers the following to be Cancer-causing:

- **60%** of all herbicides – weed killers.
- **90%** of all fungicides – which kill, you guessed it, the fungus among us.
- **30%** of all insecticides – the insect killers, obviously.

Karen: Some of these chemicals are no longer used in the US because they were found to be too toxic and a danger to our health.

Steve: But the zinger is that many of these outlawed chemicals are still being produced in the United States. They are then sold to other countries that, in turn, ship their fruits and vegetables back to the United States! That's a bunch of ship if you ask me. Chalk up another reason to buy local!

Karen: Absolutely. When you ingest these chemicals, they accumulate in your fat cells. Over time, this toxicity can alter your genetic makeup, mimic hormones, and lead to Cancer. They affect not only our nervous system, but reproductive system as well, causing infertility in both men and women.

Steve: Okay, let's talk cost for a minute. It's the obvious thing on most people's mind when they think about organic food. Yes, organic foods tend to cost more, but here's your strategy move. The Environmental Working Group (EWG) has compiled a list of the "Dirty Dozen" … the twelve most heavily contaminated types of produce. The list is updated yearly. When it comes to the fruits and vegetables on the "Dirty Dozen" list, you really should buy organic. This is true even if it means trimming the beer budget. Okay, so here they are … the most heavily sprayed fruits and vegetables. In the number one position of most heavily sprayed are apples!

1. Apple
2. Bell Peppers
3. Blue Berries (domestic)
4. Celery
5. Cucumbers
6. Grapes
7. Lettuce
8. Nectarines (imported)
9. Peaches
10. Potatoes
11. Spinach
12. Strawberries

Karen: On the flip side, here's a list of the "Clean 15," those with the lowest pesticides. In the number one position with the least amount of pesticides is asparagus!

1. Asparagus
2. Avocado
3. Cabbage
4. Cantaloupe (domestic)
5. Corn
6. Eggplant
7. Grapefruit
8. Kiwi
9. Mangoes
10. Mushrooms
11. Onions
12. Pineapples
13. Sweat Peas
14. Sweet Potatoes
15. Watermelon

Steve: Our suggestion is to download the EWG's pocket-size cheat sheet shopping guide so you can carry it with you to the grocery store.

Karen: You can visit my website at KarenRothNutrition. com and click on the Resources tab where you'll find a link to the list under "Shopping Guides."

Steve: Remember to check back yearly because the list gets updated due to the wacky changes in our world. Okay, now that we're all on the same page about what pesticides can do to us, let's talk about food labeling... another one of Karen's obsessions ... I mean, specialties. For the record, she just shot me a look.

Karen: When you see food that's labeled "100% Organic," it means that the product is made of 100% organic ingredients. If it is a fruit or vegetable, this means that it is grown without synthetic pesticides or chemical fertilizers, does not contain genetically modified organisms, and is not processed using irradiation, industrial solvents, or chemical food additives. However, if the food package says "Organic," that means the product contains at least 95-99% organic ingredients.

Steve: See? I told you guys she was good at this. Wait, it gets better.

Karen: Food packaging that states "Made with Organic Ingredients" must contain at least 70% organic ingredients but may contain up to 94%. These products can't carry the organic seal; instead, they may list up to three organic ingredients on the front of the packaging. Products with less than 70% organic ingredients may only list "Organic Ingredients" on the information panel of the packaging. These products will not bear the USDA organic seal.

Steve: Tell them about the PLU code. You guys are going to like this one. Inside scoop.

Karen: PLU is the abbreviation for "Price Look Up." You find these tiny stickers on your fruits and vegetables, and they tell you if the fruit was organically grown or produced with chemical fertilizers, fungicides, or herbicides. Here's how to read the PLU code:

- Fruits and veggies conventionally grown have four numbers ... such as 1234.
- Organic fruits and veggies have a "9" before it ... such as 91234.

Steve: I love this inside stuff. It's not only great "I know more than you" information to share at your poker game, but it makes you an informed consumer.

Karen: Bottom line, gentlemen ...

Steve: Wait. You did the bottom line in the last chapter.

Karen: Fine. Go ahead.

Steve: Just protecting the herd. Can't have you calling them "gentlemen" more than I call them "guys" or they may actually start to believe they're gentlemen.

Karen: Heaven forbid that should happen.

Steve: Oh, I agree. **Here's the bottom line, CAVEMEN. Know what you're eating, and eat organic whenever possible, especially the fruits and vegetables listed as the "Dirty Dozen."**

Does Your Meat Roll in the Grass?

Steve: I just love the name of this chapter.

Karen: Now there's a surprise.

Steve: Guys can relate to this kind of humor. And since this book was written with guys in mind, it's highly appropriate.

Karen: Not everyone shares your sense of humor.

Steve: I would venture to say most of our male readers do. The others are eating too much soy.

Karen: Okay, I have a confession to make. I do like the name of this chapter.

Steve: I knew it!

Karen: I like my beef coming from cows that enjoy the wide open spaces … prancing up and down hillsides … lounging under trees on the range…lying down in the wide open fields when they're tired. Wild and free!

Steve: Surprised you didn't say "dancing."

Karen: Cows don't dance.

Steve: Enough of this, let's get to the meat of this section. When it comes to shopping, some people shop for meat either by what's on sale or by what looks good. You know, the way college guys do 30 minutes before the bar closes.

Karen: I can't believe you went there.

Steve: Guy readers, remember? And what's important to keep in mind when it comes to buying steaks, ribs, and roasts is that there is a big difference between grass-fed, hormone-free beef, and everything that's not.

Karen: Cattle raised on commercial feedlots are fed grains (mostly corn) and typically have to be administered antibiotics daily on this type of diet. In addition they are given growth hormones to cause rapid weight gain.

Steve: Here are the facts. Your turn.

Karen: Compared with grain-fed beef, grass-fed beef is lower in saturated fat and higher in beneficial omega-3 fatty acids. In fact, grass-fed beef contains more omega-3s than farm raised salmon. Now there's something else called conjugated linoleic acid (CLA) which helps promote fat loss, reduce oxidative stress, decrease inflammation, and even suppresses tumor growth. Grass-fed beef is the richest known source of CLA you can get, so eating grass-fed beef rules.

Steve: It's important to always remember that the chemicals a cow eats settle in their fat. And since some of the beef you eat is fat, no matter how good a trimmer you may be ...

Karen: Even with the nose hair trimmers.

Steve: Women included. Anyway, if you eat any fat, you're ingesting all those chemicals which can affect your metabolism, mess with your fertility, and play games with your nervous system.

Karen: That's why we eat grass-fed beef that's hormone and antibiotic-free and raised on organic grasses.

Steve: Sure, grass-fed beef can sometimes cost a bit more, but c'mon ... it's your health we're talking about.

Karen: We regularly buy our organic free-range chicken and grass-fed beef at both our local farmers market and through reliable meat producers who ship directly to our house. You can find the meat producers we use under "Karen's Selections" at IMarriedaNutritionist.com.

Steve: Or check with your local grocery store or butcher. As a footnote, when buying chicken, go organic, free-range.

Karen: Agreed.

Steve: Bottom line, guys ...

Karen: My turn, remember? **Bottom line gentlemen, whenever possible, buy beef that's grass-fed, and hormone-free.**

Steve: Yep. Guys, keep your meat clean.

Karen: You just ruined my bottom line.

Steve: Sorry. I thought this topic gave me free range.

Karen: Oh brother.

Eggs – Nothing to Yoke About

Steve: When I was a kid, I wouldn't eat eggs. Reason being, they looked gross and they came from chicken butts, or somewhere down there. When I was a Boy Scout, I stomached eggs on campouts because there was lots of ketchup, and nothing else to eat for breakfast.

Karen: Yes, and it wasn't until you married a nutritionist that you truly understood what a great food source eggs were and that, if prepared right, eggs can be delicious.

Steve: Yes, they can. And yes you do get credit for me eating eggs.

Karen: Credit accepted.

Steve: Credit deserved.

Karen: Credit deserved … accepted.

Steve: Man, she's good at that. Okay, guys. There's a lot of misinformation out there about eggs. Many people avoid them or limit eating them because they think eggs will send their cholesterol through the roof. Although egg yolks are high in cholesterol, and health experts in the past have told patients with cholesterol problems to avoid this food, nutrition experts, like my nutritionist here, suggest that eating an egg a day is no problem for the majority of the population.

Karen: Absolutely. Eggs have been described as the perfect food. And I happen to agree.

Steve: She agrees … and I agree, too. Scrap the chicken butt stuff. Eggs rock!

Karen: There is, however, a *small* percentage of the population that is affected by dietary intake of cholesterol. If you're one of those people, you may want to stick with the egg whites.

Steve: Precisely. See? By saying "precisely" that lets me ride on her authoritative coattails, making me look, well, in the know. You might want to use that strategy at work. When the boss says something important, raise your finger (not your middle finger but your index finger) and say, "Precisely."

Karen: Precisely. Here are some other key things you gentlemen need to know about eggs:

- Eggs are one of the highest quality sources of proteins you can eat.
- Eggs contain choline, which promotes brain health.
- Egg whites contain loads of essential amino acids.
- Egg yolks contains lutein which is an important nutrient for the eyes.
- Eggs are one of few foods that contain vitamin D which stimulates the absorption of calcium. Great for strengthening your bones.
- Eggs are a good source of vitamin K, which anchors calcium inside the bones.
- Eggs are around 70 calories each.
- Eggs contain iodine and selenium, both critical nutrients for the thyroid.

Steve: Yep, and when it comes to hormones in eggs, run the other way. Well, not literally. Just grab an organic carton.

Karen: Buy pasture-raised, organic eggs whenever possible. Why? It's simply because non-organic chickens are often given antibiotics, which are then passed on to humans when you eat their eggs. Those antibiotics can contribute to antibiotic-resistant bacteria in humans.

Steve: Okay, let's switch gears. Brown or white eggs?

Karen: The reality is that they both have the same nutrients; they just come from different breeds of chicken.

Steve: No kidding? You never told me that.

Karen: You never asked.

Steve: You can volunteer the information.

Karen: That wouldn't be any fun.

Steve: Bottom line, guys. Eggs are a good food. Eat 'em up.

Think Twice about Holding Back Your Nuts

Steve: Okay, I know what you guys are thinking and that's not what this chapter is about.

Karen: Not fair.

Steve: What?

Karen: The title. You're leading the readers on to think one thing, and then zoom, you reverse course making them feel like they're the ones with dirty minds.

Steve: That's what guys do to each other. It's part of our communication.

Karen: Oh really?

Steve: All the time. It builds character.

Karen: Wow. I didn't know that.

Steve: Men are not simple creatures.

Karen: Apparently not.

Steve: The head nod thing? Silent communication. Back slap? Physical communication.

Karen: How about hugging when you greet each other?

Steve: Hugging? That's not hugging.

Karen: Then what is it?

Steve: We're frisking each other for weapons.

Karen: Oh brother.

Steve: Okay, guys … let's talk nuts … the kind you eat. I'm sure you've heard a lot about how some nuts may be good for you and some may be bad for you, and we're going to set the record straight. The right nuts, in the right amount, can be amazingly good for you.

Karen: The right amount is a small portion in the palm of your hand. Not a fist-full.

Steve: Precisely. A recent Spanish study showed that nuts help fight obesity and high blood pressure in those who added the snack to a high-veggie, high-fruit diet.

Karen: And for those who don't eat a lot of veggies and fruits, nuts can still make a big difference in your health. Pistachio nuts, for example, reduce triglycerides and body weight.

Steve: I did know that because … I'm married to a nutritionist. And walnuts are excellent for helping ward off coronary heart disease. They're a great source of omega 3 fatty acids which provide anti-inflammatory effects.

Karen: As for almonds, they're said to be one of the healthiest of all nuts. Why? To start, almonds have loads of calcium, heart-healthy fat, and vitamin E.

Steve: Then there's one of my favorites, macadamia nuts, which immediately makes you think of Hawaii. Either you brought them back to your friends on the mainland, or you received them from your very tan friends. Either way, macadamia nuts have some of the highest amount of good fats among all nuts.

Karen: Most of the fat in macadamia nuts is monounsaturated, which studies have shown positively affect LDL and HDL cholesterol, and lower total cholesterol.

Steve: And then there's peanuts, something most guys should know about. They have their health benefits, too.

Karen: Just avoid sucking on peanut shells at the ballgame. They're coated with a load of salt.

Steve: But sucking on peanut shells until your lips are trashed is part of the American sporting experience.

Karen: Well, I suggest you skip that part. That much salt plays havoc with your system.

Steve: Enjoying a handful of unsalted peanuts can actually give you a fair amount of fiber and protein. Now, if your nuts are raw … you better see a doctor.

Karen: Wow. For a moment, I actually thought you were going to make it through this nuts chapter without going there.

Steve: Where?

Karen: The Low Road.

Steve: Guys love the Low Road.

Karen: Part of the communication thing?

Steve: Absolutely. Now let me just say this about raw nuts. They're better for you. Roasting exposes nuts to very high temperatures, which can ruin some of the health benefits, and the extreme heat can damage the oils and create free radicals. Was that better?

Karen: Yes.

Steve: And if you insist on eating a lot of roasted nuts, consider roasting them yourself at home. Simply preheat your oven to 160 degrees, lay your nuts on a cookie sheet, and roast them for 15-20 minutes.

Karen: Why are you looking at me?

Steve: "Lay your nuts on the cookie sheet" didn't bother you?

Karen: They're your nuts.

Steve: You're tricky sometimes.

Karen: It's a woman's prerogative to be tricky.

Steve: And finally … aside from putting your nuts in your hand, nuts are a good addition to salads, cooked greens, yogurt, and oatmeal. I think I'm done.

Karen: Thank goodness. **Bottom line, gentlemen. Your nuts are your friends.**

Gluten Tooten & Quinoa

Steve: Before we begin this section I just want to say that the only reason I used "tooten" in the title was that it rhymed with gluten.

Karen: Not because gluten can cause stomach upset?

Steve: No.

Karen: And stomach upset can cause gas?

Steve: No. I mean, yes it can cause gas but no I didn't intend for "tooten" to reflect that.

Karen: Let the record show Steve has refrained from going down the path of a potential fart joke.

Steve: Okay, it was intentional. I just didn't want to get a reputation for taking the low road.

Karen: I think that train has already left the station.

Steve: Okay, back to business. We've been hearing quite a lot about gluten these days.

Karen: We certainly have. Some of that news surrounds athletes who have discovered that they can compete better by removing gluten from their diets.

Steve: Case in point, Serbian tennis star Novak Djokovic. A nutritionist discovered that Djokovic was allergic to gluten, and since the tennis player removed it from his diet, along with processed carbohydrates, his performance has gone through the roof.

Karen: Pretty amazing, but not surprising.

Steve: So what is gluten anyway?

Karen: Gluten is …

Steve: Wait. That was a rhetorical question. I was actually going to answer that after the dramatic pause.

Karen: Oh, is that what that was? Okay, well go ahead.

Steve: Actually, you kinda took all the drama out of it. You can go ahead and explain it.

Karen: How about I help you?

Steve: Kind of feeling left out, huh?

Karen: Go right ahead.

Steve: Gluten is a protein substance that is found in such grains as wheat, barley, and rye.

Karen: Another dramatic pause?

Steve: No, that's pretty much it.

Karen: I see.

Steve: You're the expert. I'm just the healthy spouse. I put the ball on the tee so you can drive it down the fairway.

Karen: That's very generous of you.

Steve: Well, I'm just that sort of guy.

Karen: There are a few reasons why gluten is commonly found in so many of the foods we eat. For bakers, gluten keeps the gases released during fermentation in the dough, and that allows dough to rise. Additionally, gluten helps baked goods retain their shape. As you mentioned, gluten is found in wheat, and wheat flour is in literally thousands of packaged and prepared foods. So you can understand why people who have sensitivity to gluten, such as Novak Djokovic, have challenges with what they can and can not eat.

Steve: When you have Gluten Intolerance, as millions of people do, the gluten attacks your small intestines by destroying the villi which eventually leads to the formation of tiny holes in your intestines. Why don't you tell them what villi are?

Karen: Teeing it up again?

Steve: You bet.

Karen: Villi are finger-like projections on the intestinal surface. When the villi are destroyed, and the holes are created, food particles leak into your bloodstream and are seen by your body's defense system as "foreign invaders." In the process, you lose the absorption of important nutrients as your body starts to attack itself.

Steve: So if you don't want to take a leak, or create a leak in this case, keep that villi in place.

Karen: Researchers are discovering that more and more illnesses can be tied to Gluten Intolerance. So I find that even people who aren't diagnosed with Gluten Sensitivity can benefit by cutting back or completely removing gluten from their diets.

Steve: And, today, avoiding gluten is getting easier as more and more gluten-free products are hitting the shelves. I read somewhere that 10% of all new products are gluten-free. If people demand it, manufacturers will make it.

Karen: One of our favorite substitutes for grains like wheat and barley in almost any recipe is quinoa.

Steve: Which is pronounced "Keen-Wah," not "Quinn-Noah" as I first called it. If Anthony Quinn played Noah, that movie would be called *Quinn-Noah*.

Karen: Quinoa is commonly thought of as a grain, but it's really a seed of a plant in the same family of leafy greens like Swiss chard. It has been around for thousands of years and dates back to 3000 BC.

Steve: Karen makes a killer cold quinoa salad and you can find the recipe on her website, KarenRothNutrition.com.

Karen: It's so easy to make and only takes 15 minutes to cook. Quinoa is an excellent source of iron which promotes energy production, making it a great pick-me-up food.

Steve: It also has a lot of fiber to keep you regular.

Karen: Quinoa can also lower cholesterol, and the magnesium you get from it relaxes your blood vessels, so it's heart healthy. Quinoa is also low on the Glycemic Index so it's a good choice for Diabetics.

Steve: Did you know that quinoa contains more protein than any other grain?

Karen: I did know that. And that protein is of an unusually high quality, containing all nine essential amino acids.

Steve: I kind of knew that, too.

Karen: Right.

Steve: Quinoa is really catching on with consumers and you can now find quinoa cookies, cereals, and pasta.

Karen: When cooking with quinoa, remember that 1 cup will cook up to 4 cups. And you'll always want to rinse it well before cooking. Quinoa is coated with a compound that is a natural insect repellent that, if not rinsed off, will turn soapy when cooked.

Steve: So there you have it. Everything you always wanted to know about quinoa.

Karen: As well as a good overview on gluten.

Steve: You ready?

Karen: For what?

Steve: Bottom line time.

Karen: Have at it.

Steve: Guys, the bottom line on gluten is that even if you don't have Gluten Sensitivity, you might want to cut back or eliminate it from your diet. And then, you too can become a professional tennis player!

For a boatload of healthy product suggestions, visit:
IMarriedaNutritionist.com
Click on "Karen's Selections."

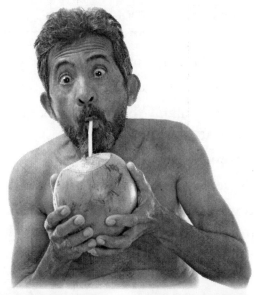

THE LIQUID STUFF

CHAPTER 2

*"I think it's liquid aggravation that circulates through his veins, and not regular blood." ~ **Charles Dickens***

*"I think Charles Dickens needs to suggest his friend drink more water to dilute that liquid aggravation in his veins." ~ **Steve Roth***

Coconut Water for
Hydration & Hangovers

Steve: Welcome to the liquid chapter.

Karen: If you can't swim, it's not an issue. Why are you looking at me?

Steve: That was pretty good.

Karen: Thank you.

Steve: I mean, usually I'm the one who says things like that.

Karen: Yes, usually. But not this time.

Steve: Hmmm. You're not thinking of making this a regular thing, are you?

Karen: What?

Steve: Saying things like "If you can't swim, it's not an issue."

Karen: Nah. Because if I said it again, I would be repeating myself, and comedy often relies on the element of surprise. Booo!

Steve: What's with you?

Karen: I don't know. I just got to thinking, here I am stuck in the role of the authority figure, and you get to say all the fun things.

Steve: Well, you can say some fun things, too.

Karen: I may just do that.

Steve: From time to time.

Karen: We'll see. What do you say we get this train moving?

Steve: We're now going to talk about something Karen turned me on to years ago … coconut water.

Karen: Yes. Coconut water is not only low in calories, it's low in fat, and it doesn't have nearly the sugar that most bottled beverages do.

Steve: And if you were awake during our sugar discussion in the first chapter, you'll remember that sugar is not your best friend.

Karen: No, it's not. And it's important to note that before you buy coconut water at the store …

Steve: … Which is available in convenient can and carton sizes … Like that announcer voice I just used?

Karen: Brilliant moment of spontaneity.

Steve: Sometimes I can't control it. The genius just happens.

Karen: That's what Einstein said. Did you know he was a relativity of mine? What? That wasn't funny?

Steve: Think authority.

Karen: Oh, you're no fun. Okay, back to the coconut water. Before buying it, check the ingredients and make sure you're getting pure coconut water, without added sugar and other ingredients.

Steve: As you may have read in the "About the Authors" section at the back of the book, I'm a competitive archer. Coconut water has turned out to be a great tool in my arsenal, especially on hot days when we're competing outside. It's an amazing hydrator.

Karen: Absolutely. Next time you're exercising, skip the sports drink and replace it with coconut water.

Steve: It's important to note that most sports drinks contain sugar and artificial colors which play havoc with your body.

Karen: Havoc? That's a strange word if you think about it. I mean, it's really not used in everyday conversation but you'll often hear it describing TV crime shows. "The Killer's on the loose, and he's creating havoc ..." Havoc. It's even spelled weird. A little too much?

Steve: Just a little.

Karen: Beyond sports, hydration plays a big role in why you feel so bad after a night of drinking. When you drink alcohol, whether it's beer, wine, or liquor, you're dehydrating your body. And when you reach that mode, your body has a hard time absorbing water.

Steve: Coconut water, which is loaded with pure and natural electrolytes, quickly puts you on the road to recovery.

Karen: And if you want to go *au naturel* ...

Steve: Score!

Karen: Then be adventurous and buy a whole coconut at the store. Poke out the soft hole on the end ... one of the three divots is always soft ... and drain out the pure juice or use a straw. But don't throw the coconut away!

Steve: Absolutely not! Tap in to your primal guy instincts and smash that sucker open with a hammer. Inside, you'll find all this delicious white coconut meat. It's a fantastic snack.

Karen: Explain to them how you separate the coconut meat from the shell.

Steve: Simple. I take a clean regular screwdriver and work the tip down between the shell and coconut meat. It takes a little practice, but once you get the rhythm it goes pretty quickly. You might want to put on music with a good beat, but avoid Barry White or you'll be there making love to your coconut for hours.

Karen: That was so random.

Steve: Yes, it was.

Karen: Bottom line, gentlemen. Pure natural coconut water outperforms sports drinks for hydration. I think we're off to a good start with this liquid chapter.

Steve: Feeling empowered?

Karen: You bet.

Steve: Then I bet and the pot's even.

Karen: I don't get it.

Steve: Poker?

Karen: Why? She didn't do anything.

Steve: What?

Karen: Poke her. Get it?

Steve: Unfortunately... yes.

The Inside Scoop on Coffee

Steve: Like most people, I've been drinking coffee first thing in the morning for more years than I care to admit. Roll out of bed, stagger to the kitchen, and pour the Joe.

Karen: Ever wonder why people call it Joe?

Steve: Because John was already taken for the toilet?

Karen: Okay, that was funny. The origins of the name Joe for coffee are still uncertain. But we do know that Joe was a nickname used for coffee in the military in the early 1900s, along with the name Java. In the 1960s, the name Joe for coffee went mainstream.

Steve: And you just happened to know that because …?

Karen: There's this thing called the Internet, and while you were blah-blah-blahing about coconut water, I did a little research knowing you would refer to coffee as Joe in this section.

Steve: That's quite impressive … and proactive.

Karen: That's my job, staying two steps ahead of you.

Steve: Okay, back to the … Java. See? I didn't say Joe. Whether you brew your coffee in some cheap plastic machine that leaks, or in a nice coffeemaker from Macy's that you got for your wedding, or you go all fancy on us and use a French press or drip filter, it all gets us to the same place … morning buzz pick-me-up before hitting the shower.

Karen: It's a morning routine for many people.

Steve: It wasn't too long ago that Karen started making hot cocoa sweetened with stevia, leaving all the morning coffee to me. As much as the hot cocoa smelled good, I wasn't about to give up my morning jolt. No way.

Karen: Then he finally listened to what I had to say about drinking coffee first thing in the morning on an empty stomach.

Steve: Do continue.

Karen: In Stephen Cherniske's book titled *Caffeine Blues,* he points out that caffeine, especially on an empty stomach, stimulates the adrenal glands to produce cortisol … the body's foremost stress hormone that also stores fat.

Steve: And that's when I sensed danger, Will Robinson.

Karen: Chronic long-term exposure to stress hormones disrupts the body's metabolism, causing elevated blood sugar, high cholesterol, high blood pressure, and increased fat levels due to increased appetite. Stress makes you burn fewer calories, and cortisol can actually reduce the body's ability to release fat from its fat stores to use for energy.

Steve: And that's when it hit me. I may be getting fat by drinking my morning coffee.

Karen: Now, in defense of coffee, studies have shown that coffee drinkers are less likely to have Type 2 Diabetes, Parkinson's Disease, and Dementia … along with fewer cases of heart rhythm problems and Strokes. And new research indicates that women who drink lots of coffee, at least four cups a day, are 25% less likely to develop Endometrial Cancer than women who don't finish one cup.

Steve: That's good news for Starbucks.

Karen: There's also increasing evidence that Prostate Cancer doesn't like coffee, both leaded and decaf, if you drink one to six cups a day.

Steve: Okay, now you're talking.

Karen: Get this. Three cups of coffee a day, according to research, also helps shut down Basal Cell Carcinoma.

Steve: Can you pass the coffee pot, please?

Karen: Finally, the latest research shows that women who drink lots of coffee, at least five cups a day of regular, also run a lower risk of certain types of Breast Cancer after menopause ... 20% to 50% lower versus women who have less than one cup a day.

Steve: So, to sum things up ... to minimize my getting fat ...

Karen: Fatter ...

Steve: ... I now drink cocoa instead of coffee, on an empty stomach. Then drink coffee other times of the day. Plus, cocoa in the morning is a great waker-upper without all the amped-up caffeine feeling.

Karen: And there's a reason it feels good to drink cocoa in the morning. Unlike coffee, which can be fat-storing on an empty stomach, cocoa is a fat-burning food. Plus, cocoa has the ability to directly affect the pleasure centers in your brain, making you feel satisfied, motivated, and energized.

Steve: Just make sure you use only 100% unsweetened, non-dairy Baker's Cocoa Powder.

Karen: Yes, and sweeten it with stevia, or even xylitol.

Steve: Bottom line, guys. **Caffeine on an empty stomach may be making you fat. Coffee, at other times, may promote good health.**

Cranberry Juice
Beyond Shirt Stains

Steve: Ah, yes. Cranberries … nature's little floating berry that packs a punch when it comes to health benefits. It's also a nice mixer with vodka.

Karen: Yes it is.

Steve: Like a lot of people, Karen and I enjoy wine and cocktails, and certainly a lot of terrific food. We just try to go about it in a way that benefits us the most and does as little wear and tear on the body as possible. Correcto?

Karen: If you say so.

Steve: And since I did just say so, it's correcto!

Karen: Cranberries contain 5-times more antioxidants than broccoli and may prevent Kidney Stones and Urinary Tract Infections. The phytonutrients may protect against Macular Degeneration.

Steve: Yep, gotta protect the eyes.

Karen: Heart issues are a main topic of conversation these days, and it's good to know that drinking cranberry juice or eating the whole cranberry benefits the heart. Research shows that cranberries lower LDL cholesterol while kicking up the good HDL.

Steve: Now before you run down to the store to load up on Cranberry Juice Cocktail, Karen suggests sticking with 100% pure cranberry juice to reap the most benefits. You will also avoid the extra sugar from the juices, like grape juice, that they add to make it sweet.

Karen: There are a lot of cranberry juices to choose from, but don't be fooled by "light" or "sugar-free" labeling because those drinks usually contain artificial sweeteners. Again, you want 100% no–sugar–added cranberry juice. If it's not sweet enough for you, you can always add a touch of stevia or xylitol, which you learned about in the Sugar Chapter.

Steve: Okay, now for a little trivia. When cranberry fields are harvested, they flood the fields and drive a machine through the water that shakes the bushes below. Whala, the cranberries float to the top like bubbles streaming out of a farting kid's bathing suit.

Karen: I think we're done with cranberries.

Steve: It was the fart thing, right?

Karen: Bottom line, gentlemen. Cranberry juice promotes good health, but stick with 100% juice with no added sugar.

Steve: Absolutely. And back to the floating berry thing. The reason why cranberries float is that they have little air chambers inside. It has just enough air to bring it to the surface.

Karen: Like a kid who farts in his bathing suit?

Steve: That would have to be a very big fart to bring him to the surface.

Karen: We're done.

Resveratrol – Hard to Say but Worth Learning

Steve: Okay, here's one of those big picture tips I've learned from Karen which can potentially extend your life in a major way. Get to know Resveratrol (pronounced: rez-vir-a-trol).

Karen: Absolutely. Resveratrol is a phytonutrient found in the skin of grapes, grape juice, berries, and red wine, and it's often been recommended for its life-extending properties. Phytonutrients, also known has phytochemicals, are specific health-promoting substances found in plant food. Resveratrol is a powerful antioxidant that may help prevent Cancer, cut inflammation, lower cholesterol, and may lower the risk of Colon Cancer. If you know of someone with Alzheimer's Disease, studies indicate it may slow its progression.

Steve: Now you see why it's worth learning the word? It also scores a lot of points in Scrabble.

Karen: New studies have shown that resveratrol also has the potential to help with weight-loss and can kick up your metabolism.

Steve: It even helps with blood flow through the body by opening blood vessels, and guys, you know what that means. Can't guarantee you'll be walking down the hall at work with a binder in front of your belt buckle, but you may be pitching more tents, more often without going camping!

Karen: Are we in fifth grade?

Steve: No, I think it was more like first year of junior high school.

Karen: Gentlemen, if your wife is dealing with symptoms of menopause and you're reeling from the effects, a new study revealed that resveratrol may be just as effective as HRT (hormone replacement therapy) in cutting symptoms of menopause without the Cancer risks!

Steve: Now if you drink a boat load of wine every day to get your resveratrol, well, you might feel good, except in the morning, but that's counterproductive. And it's hard to down so much grape juice on a regular basis. So, here's our tip. You want to tell them or should I?

Karen: You're doing so well, I hate to stop an out of control train.

Steve: Not out of control, I'm just expressing my enthusiasm for the subject!

Karen: Is that what that is? Hmmm. You can get resveratrol in a highly concentrated form and take it as a supplement the way Steve and I do.

Steve: Bottom line, guys, no matter where you get your resveratrol ... from grapes, berries, red wine, or a supplement, it packs a serious punch and promotes good health in a major way.

Beyond the Burp
Carbonated Beverages

Steve: I can't tell you how many people I know who drink carbonated soda on a daily basis.

Karen: Since you don't know the exact number, perhaps this will help. According to the Beverage Marketing Corporation, the average American consumes 44.7 gallons of soda each year. A lot of that is being ingested by children.

Steve: That's some serious soda guzzling!

Karen: Tell me about it. Like smoking, people are aware that drinking many name-brand carbonated sodas on a regular basis is not healthy for them, yet they do it anyway. Some have the ability to cut back but don't want to, others just don't care.

Steve: And for some, they are literally addicted to the caffeine, much the way heavy coffee drinkers are.

Karen: That's true.

Steve: One of the main problems with consuming soda is sugar and artificial sweeteners, correcto?

Karen: Correcto. One 12-ounce can of soda has 10 teaspoons of sugar. As we learned in an earlier chapter, research shows that sugar can cause your body to retain fluid, causes headaches and migraines, reduces learning capacity, causes depression, is addictive, and can be intoxicating, similar to alcohol. If you are coming down with something or already have become sick, the worst thing you can do is eat or drink sugar.

Steve: You didn't mention weight gain.

Karen: Well, that's a given. Here's another problem many people don't know about drinking soda.

Steve: Perhaps it's time to sound the "Inside Scoop" alarm.

Karen: Please do. Many people who try to avoid sugar, instead reach for the diet soda, some of which contain a whopping 180 milligrams of aspartame per 12-ounce can.

Steve: And earlier we explained that aspartame converts in your system to methanol.

Karen: And here's more bad news. When methanol, an alcohol, breaks down in the body, it becomes formaldehyde.

Steve: So that's why so many restaurants choose to put it on their tables. The formaldehyde preserves their customer base!

Karen: That was a good one. As you may be aware, many American soda brands are sweetened with high-fructose corn syrup, which is a man-made compound derived from genetically engineered corn.

Steve: And the problem with that is …? I'm teeing it up for you.

Karen: By consuming genetically modified foods, otherwise known as GMOs, you're essentially becoming a lab rat.

Steve: Now we're not saying you'll grow a tail … we think … but you will become a part of a long-term global experiment.

Karen: Exactly. Genetically engineered foods have only been in our food chain since the 1990s, and no one knows the long-term health impacts of eating GMOs. The corporations that developed these crops never had to test them for long-term safety.

Steve: Dude, that's not good.

Karen: Dude?

Steve: Sorry. Dudette.

Karen: The last thing I'm going to say about genetically engineered crops is that recent findings suggest that GMOs may be linked to digestive tract damage, accelerated aging, and even infertility.

Steve: There's a big movement going on right now to force food manufactures to list on labels when GMO ingredients are used.

Karen: Look for it. It'll be coming to your state.

Steve: Honestly, I don't know why food manufacturers are so worried about listing GMOs on their labels.

Karen: Isn't it obvious?

Steve: Well, if you think about it, cigarette manufacturers were forced to put a warning label on their products, and I'm guessing it didn't affect sales very much.

Karen: However, it at least provided the consumer the right to know the risks involved in what they're putting in their bodies. Nothing was hidden.

Steve: I think they should have used a more thought-provoking warning on cigarettes.

Karen: Oh, really?

Steve: Yep. "Keep smoking. We need to thin out the herd." That would have gotten attention.

Karen: You're probably right. Okay, we're getting off track. This section is about carbonated beverages.

Steve: Yes, it is. Bubble on.

Karen: Putting sweeteners aside, most brands of soft drinks are very high in phosphate. For a long time, soft drinks have been suspected of causing low levels of calcium and high levels of phosphate in the blood. The problem here is that when your calcium levels are low and phosphate levels are high, your body literally pulls calcium out of your bones making them weaker.

Steve: And I'm guessing that could lead to things like Osteoporosis.

Karen: Among other things.

Steve: Yep. One thing guys don't want is weak bones.

Karen: Or women for that matter.

Steve: And I just love this one. Some brands of soda use brominated vegetable oil — a toxic flame retardant — to keep the citrus flavorings from separating from the rest of the liquid.

Karen: Brominated vegetable oil will often be listed in soda and sports drink ingredients as BVO. BVO can cause bromide poisoning symptoms such as memory loss, nerve disorders, and skin lesions.

Steve: Okay, I think we've made our point. Now, what are healthier options for people who love to drink soda?

Karen: Well, the good news is, due to consumer demand, a number of beverage manufacturers are now making truly healthy sodas.

Steve: Healthy as in using stevia and other natural sweeteners and ingredients?

Karen: Exactly. There are many great carbonated beverages on the market that are naturally sweetened with stevia, xylitol, and/or erythritol.

Steve: For our healthy beverage recommendations, visit the "Karen's Selections" tab at IMarriedaNutritionist.com.

Karen: Bottom line, gentlemen. When it comes to sodas, it's best to avoid the ones with sugar, artificial sweeteners, and unnatural ingredients.

Taking the E Out of
Energy Drinks ... Nergy

Steve: Now we're going to talk about something that is a thorn in my nutritionist's side. Energy drinks.

Karen: Yes, we're going to remove the E from Energy.

Steve: Which leaves us with Nergy, a made-up word that sounds as silly as traditional energy drinks themselves.

Karen: Just like most carbonated beverages such as soda, many traditional energy drinks offer your body little in the way of nutrition. There may be some B vitamins in some drinks, as well as some amino acids, but that's certainly overshadowed by the effects of sugar and caffeine.

Steve: Starting off with sugar-free energy drinks, let's take a look at some of the ingredients you may find inside.

Karen: First up is acesulfame potassium, which we mentioned earlier. Remember the Ace-K abbreviation? Second up is sucralose, which is chlorinated artificial sugar that has been found to cause tumors in animals.

Steve: Splenda anyone? You know that one! It's a brand name for a sucralose-based artificial sweetener.

Karen: You may also find aspartame in energy drinks. This artificial sweetener has been linked to brain damage and brain tumors in animals and it's not recommended for growing children. You can also find artificial flavors and colorings in many brands of energy drinks.

Steve: Some energy drinks even disguise their two-serving can by advertising it as "Double Strength!"

Karen: With two-serving cans, it could mean you're consuming somewhere in the neighborhood of 200 calories, along with 44 grams of sugar or the equivalent of 11 teaspoons of sugar. The 160 milligrams or so of caffeine content isn't even as much as a small Starbucks black coffee. Makes you wonder where the energy is coming from.

Steve: Pass the sugar.

Karen: How about we not?

Steve: What about sodium? Is that something people have to worry about in many energy drinks?

Karen: You bet. Many energy drinks have around 360 milligrams of sodium in each can. A common ingredient is also high fructose corn syrup, which is known to disrupt insulin levels, and can raise your triglycerides.

Steve: This must be getting depressing for energy drink drinkers.

Karen: Many energy drinks also contain sodium benzoate. This is a chemical preservative that can cause intestinal upset and should be avoided by people with impaired liver function. Artificial colorings are commonly used in energy drinks. Yellow Dye #5, for example, is an artificial color that is required by law to be listed on food packaging because so many people are allergic to it. People with asthma and people sensitive to aspirin can react very badly to Yellow Dye #5. It's no wonder the dye is banned in Norway and Austria.

Steve: Bottom line, guys. If you're looking for an energy kick, you might want to consider healthier alternatives such as coconut water, coffee, tea, or some of the new healthy-ingredient energy drinks, with natural ingredients, which have recently hit the market. For our favorite drinks, check out "Karen's Selections" at IMarriedaNutritionist.com.

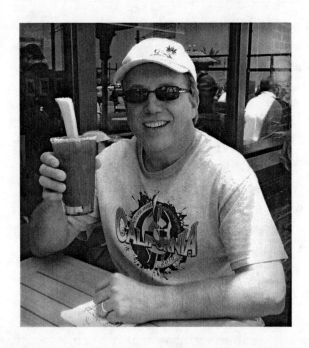

Oh Yeah! A Healthy Bloody Mary Mix!

Steve: We're going to end this chapter on liquids with a recipe for a healthy Bloody Mary mix.

Karen: One of my favorites.

Steve: Yep. Nothing like a fresh, home-made Bloody Mary to kick off a weekend morning. If you find yourself consuming Bloody Marys at work, instead of coffee, you either have a really cool office or you're pushing the "they won't fire me" envelope.

Karen: Most store-bought Bloody Mary mixes tend to be loaded with salt, sugar, preservatives, and all sorts of crap.

Steve: Hey! Did you just say "crap" in our book?

Karen: I don't know. Did I?

Steve: You did.

Karen: Is that a problem?

Steve: Well, no … it was just a bit unexpected.

Karen: But aren't you the one always calling me the Practical Nutritionist, one who promotes health and nutrition in a way that's down to earth and easy to understand?

Steve: Yes.

Karen: And one who says what's on her mind?

Steve: Yes.

Karen: Well, what was on my mind is that a lot of Bloody Mary mixes are loaded with crap.

Steve: Boy, you're getting a bit feisty.

Karen: It's a woman's prerogative.

Steve: Ooooookay.

Karen: In my opinion, some store-bought Bloody Mary mixes are fine in a pinch. Read the label and find the healthiest one you can. But if you have the time, why not make it from scratch so you can control what goes in your cake hole.

Steve: Cake hole? Did I just hear that from you?

Karen: Prerogative, remember?

Steve: I want to do the prerogative thing.

Karen: You always do, you just don't know it.

Steve: You're right. I think.

Karen: Home-made Bloody Marys taste like no other, whether you make them yourself or you find a restaurant that whips them up from scratch.

Steve: Like the one I'm enjoying in the photo at The Lighthouse Cafe in Hermosa Beach. Believe me, there's a reason that celery stick was so erect. It was happy to be home-made.

Karen: Home-made Bloody Marys are also good for you.

The vitamin C you get can actually counteract the free radical damage caused from the vodka. This way, you're back to even and maybe even ahead of the game.

Steve: Unless you're a lush.

Karen: Here's an example of a terrific home-made Bloody Mary Mix recipe.

- 3 tablespoons Dijon mustard
- 3 tablespoons Worcestershire sauce
- 2 tablespoons horseradish
- 2 tablespoons hot sauce
- 1 teaspoon celery seed
- 2 lemons juiced
- 2 limes juiced
- 2 teaspoons fresh ground black pepper
- 2 teaspoons sea salt

Mix all of the above ingredients together. Next, begin to add the mix to 8 cups of low- sodium tomato juice to taste, depending on how spicy you prefer.

Steve: Let's take a closer look at some of those ingredients.

Karen: Tomato Juice contains vitamins A and C, which help fight inflammation. Lemons and limes have high levels of vitamin C to fight free radicals and strengthen the immune system. Horseradish helps protect against food-borne illnesses, such as Listeria, E. Coli, and Staphylococcus. It also promotes a healthy gallbladder, improves digestion, and helps us digest fats and oils.

Steve: Hot sauce helps burn more calories by boosting your metabolic rate.

Karen: Yes, and celery is high in potassium, helps lower blood pressure and it's a natural diuretic. Works like a broom to sweep out your digestive track, getting rid of toxins and cholesterol, and it's a natural detoxifier.

Steve: You know, I think I'm going to go get healthy and make myself a Bloody Mary.

Karen: Maybe you should, right after you make me one.

Steve: That's so practical of you.

Karen: I know, I try.

Steve: Bottom line, guys. Bloody Marys can be good for you if they include the right ingredients. Try making your own from scratch! It's the best kind. See you in the next chapter.

For a boatload of healthy product suggestions, visit:
IMarriedaNutritionist.com
Click on "Karen's Selections."

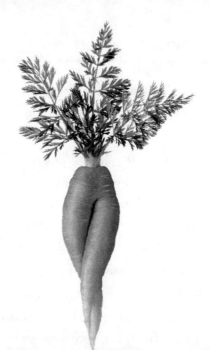

THE VEGGIE STUFF

CHAPTER 3

*"Imagination is the real and eternal world of which this vegetable universe is but a faint shadow." ~ **William Blake***

"I'm thinking William Blake had one too many Bloody Mary's for breakfast." ~ Steve Roth

Headline: Killer Artie Chokes Three for a Dollar

Steve: The globe artichoke is one the world's oldest cultivated vegetables.

Karen: You're such a fountain of knowledge.

Steve: And my fountain overfloweth. Did you know that in the US, 99% of all globe artichokes are grown right here in California?

Karen: No, I didn't know that. Did you know that globe artichokes are very low in calories at only 60 calories per artichoke?

Steve: I did know that. Okay, I didn't know that.

Karen: Most of the carbohydrates you find in artichokes are in the form of inulin, which makes this a very beneficial vegetable to add to your diet — especially if you're Diabetic. Inulin has been shown to improve blood sugar in Diabetics.

Steve: Now look who's a fountain of knowledge.

Karen: Artichokes are also an excellent source of fiber, magnesium, and chromium. The chromium, in particular, provides another benefit to Diabetics, since it improves blood sugar levels. Artichokes also contain iodine, which is essential for fat metabolism and thyroid function.

Steve: Okay, now let's talk about how you choose the right artichoke at the store.

Karen: You want to look for one that is heavy for its size and make sure the leaves are tightly compacted. You also want to look at the bottom of the stem. If you see small holes, that means there is worm damage.

Steve: Avoid artichokes whose leaves are either wilted, black, or have dark spots on them, you know, like an older person's hands. What are those spots, anyway?

Karen: Age spots. As we age, our skin is subjected to more and more sun damage on the hands, face, and body.

Steve: I think I have one of those right here.

Karen: That's dirt.

Steve: Phew. That was a close one!

Karen: Okay, back to the artichokes. If you squeeze the artichoke and it sounds squeaky, that means it's fresh. When you get them home, make sure to cook them within 4 days because they're highly perishable.

Steve: Didn't know that.

Karen: That's why it's so important to pick out a fresh one at the store.

Steve: Now, preparing artichokes can be a bit tricky.

Karen: Not really. You just need to know how to do it.

Steve: Which means if you don't know how to do it … it's tricky.

Karen: But after reading this, everyone will know, and therefore it won't be tricky.

Steve: That was a tricky way to explain it. You're tricky, you know that?

Karen: To prepare your artichoke for cooking, first rinse it well under cold water and gently scrub the leaves with a soft kitchen brush. With a sharp knife, cut about one inch from the top of the artichoke, then remove the stem by cutting it flush with the bottom.

Steve: And now comes the cooking.

Karen: The easiest way to prepare artichokes is to steam them. Place them in a large steamer, stem down and leaves up, and steam them in about an inch of water. If you add lemon juice to the water, that will keep the artichoke from darkening. Depending on the size of the artichoke, it can take 25–40 minutes to cook. You'll know they're done when the leaves around the stem are easy to pull off.

Steve: Now, for people who have never eaten an artichoke, you don't eat the whole leaf. That would be some serious roughage.

Karen: If you could even chew it.

Steve: What you want to do is put a leaf between your teeth, with the meaty stem end inside your mouth, and gently pull it out. Your teeth will remove the meat. It seems like a lot of work for a little bit of artichoke meat, but consider this step the appetizer.

Karen: Absolutely. After you've gone through the leaves, you get to the heart of the artichoke, which is the base of the stem. Using a sharp knife, you cut out the hair-like fibers, leaving a nicely trimmed artichoke heart.

Steve: Now, if you're thinking about removing the hair-like fibers by waxing …

Karen: Don't go there.

Steve: Just wanted to see if you were listening.

Karen: Some people like to dip their artichoke leaves in garlic butter or lemon mayonnaise. If you're watching calories, then opt for plain yogurt mixed with lemon juice and garlic, or just dip the leaves in some balsamic vinaigrette.

Steve: I go with the garlic in melted butter. And I use real butter, not margarine. Despite its reputation, real butter is something your system recognizes.

Karen: And on a totally different note, if artichokes are left to bloom, they can grow up to 5 feet tall. When they bloom, they produce the most beautiful flower. You can find blooming artichokes for decoration purposes at your local farmer's market, and I've actually found them at our grocery store in the floral department.

Steve: Bottom line, guys. Artichokes are a pretty cool, healthy, and tasty food. Serve them up, and you'll impress your wife, girlfriend, friends, but maybe not the guys at your next poker game.

Asparagus – The Stinky Pee Vegetable

Steve: Many years back when Karen and I were first dating, she would cook amazing meals for me that often included asparagus. Up until that time, I wasn't a big asparagus fan because when I was growing up, my mother always over-cooked it into mush.

Karen: And it probably came out of a can, which didn't help.

Steve: You got that right. The funny part of the story is that when Karen would make asparagus, my pee would stink. And not being a regular asparagus eater, I didn't make the connection between the stinky pee and asparagus. I thought I had something strange going on in my gut. I mean, my pee would stink so bad my eyes would water!

Karen: Then one night over dinner, Steve admits to his smelly problem.

Steve: I said something like … I think my insides are rotting out, or I'm starting to prematurely decompose.

Karen: He explained what he was experiencing with smelly urine. Of course, with asparagus being my favorite vegetable, I knew exactly what it was.

Steve: I can't tell you how relieved I was to know I wasn't dying. I think from that point on, I wore goggles in her bathroom after eating asparagus.

Karen: You did not.

Steve: Gas mask?

Karen: Hardly. You opened the window and held your breath. Did you know that there are scientific debates about this smell?

Steve: No, I didn't. Tell me more.

Karen: Depending on which study you read, between 22% and 50% of the population report pungent pee after eating asparagus. This odorous phenomenon is where the ongoing debates and theories come into play. The first theory claims that everyone's urine is in fact affected by asparagus, but only about half of the population has the specific gene that is required to smell the change. The second theory claims that only half of the world's population has the gene that's needed to break down the compounds found in asparagus and, if the body doesn't break them down, no smell is emitted.

Steve: Cool beans. I mean, asparagus.

Karen: Historically asparagus has been used as a natural remedy for sufferers of Arthritis and Rheumatism because of its antioxidant and anti-inflammatory properties.

Steve: It has also been used as a diuretic, which doesn't help with the pee smell if you get it.

Karen: Asparagus is low in calories at only 24 calories for a full cup! It's also low in carbohydrates, a rich source of protein compared to other vegetables, and also a good source of fiber.

Steve: Which keeps you regular. And guys who are regular are not as full of crap as others believe.

Karen: Oh, so you can say "crap?"

Steve: Hey, I have to catch up to you.

Karen: At the store, you want to buy asparagus with fresh dark green tips that are tightly closed and bottom stalks that are not dried out. If you aren't going to cook them right away when you get home, you can wrap the bottom stalks with a damp paper towel to store them and maintain freshness.

Steve: And you want to prepare asparagus within 2-3 days of purchasing it to make sure you're getting the most nutrients.

Karen: One of the best things I like about asparagus is how easy it is to cook. My favorite quick and easy way is to prepare asparagus by baking it. First thing you want to do is bend the bottom of each stalk so it naturally snaps off the hard part. Next, thoroughly rinse the stalks. I lay them flat in a glass Pyrex baking dish and pour coconut oil over them. Then I bake the asparagus at 400 degrees for no more than 10 minutes. At about 5 minutes, you'll want to take them out and toss them around to re-coat them evenly with the oil. Simple and delicious!

Steve: Steaming is another popular way to prepare asparagus. When it's done, you can put a little oil or butter on it and chow down. Or some people like it without anything added.

Karen: Asparagus is also terrific in stir-fries, added to pasta sauce, or another favorite of mine … adding it to scrambled eggs. You lightly sauté a couple of chopped spears with a handful of fresh or frozen spinach and it makes some killer scrambled eggs. Imagine starting your day off with two servings of vegetables with that one dish.

Steve: Asparagus is also good caveman style.

Karen: Caveman style?

Steve: Raw, baby! Forget the cooking stuff. Just chop it up into bite-size pieces and toss in a salad. Or dip them in sauce while you're watching football with the guys.

Karen: Oh, that bathroom's going to smell really good.

Steve: Well, for at least half of us!

Karen: Bottom line, gentlemen. Why just rely on your farts to clear a room when you can eat asparagus?

Steve: What?! You can't wrap up this section like that. Only I can.

Karen: Oh, so you want me to do a more prim and proper wrap-up?

Steve: Well, it doesn't have to be prim and proper but you were doing so well with the other ones.

Karen: I treaded on your territory. My apologies.

Steve: Accepted.

Karen: Bottom line, gentlemen. Asparagus, when cooked just right, is a delicious and healthy alternative to many of the traditional vegetables you may be used to eating.

Steve: Better.

Karen: … And, if you're lucky, it'll make your pee stink like gas leaking out of a 20-year-old water heater.

Steve: This book is bringing out a whole other side to you.

Karen: Yes, and I think I like it.

Just Beet It

Karen: A recent study compared the antioxidant levels of some powerful vegetables, including broccoli, spinach, carrots, celery, onions, and beets. It concluded that beets had the highest antioxidant power of them all.

Steve: Go beets!

Karen: Unfortunately, beets are usually not top of mind when you're vegetable shopping at the store.

Steve: No doubt an image problem. Dark blood-red in color with way too many leaves attached.

Karen: For some people, beets are top of mind. But I agree with you, for most people, probably not.

Steve: And I have the sneaking suspicion you're about to change that.

Karen: I'll try my best. Aside from being rich in antioxidants, beets are loaded with heart-healthy nutrients like folate, magnesium, and potassium.

Steve: I also remember you telling me that beets are a low-calorie food.

Karen: One cup of cooked beets is only 75 calories.

Steve: Which leads us to how to cook them.

Karen: You guessed it. When selecting beets, look for a deep color, a smooth skin, and a solid root. Avoid soft, bruised, or shriveled beets.

Steve: No problem there. Shrivel is one of those things guys always try to avoid.

Karen: As I was saying, soft, bruised, and shriveled beets will be tough to eat and have fewer nutrients.

Steve: Now the cooking?

Karen: Almost. The key to storing beets once you get them home is to cut off the stems, put the beets in an airtight container, and store them in the refrigerator without rinsing.

Steve: Dirty beets, done dirt cheap. Dirty beets, done dirty cheap.

Karen: A little AC/DC. Very nice.

Steve: Thank you. I just channeled the lead singer.

Karen: When cooking ...

Steve: The cooking!

Karen: Why are you so excited about how to cook beets?

Steve: You know, I'm not really sure.

Karen: When cooking beets, you want to leave the skin on but chop the leaves off a few inches up from the beet. Now, you may want to use plastic gloves or cover your hands with plastic baggies to avoid staining your nails and hands.

Steve: Good tip. I don't want these guys showing up on poker night with red fingernails.

Karen: Yes, that would be a crisis, wouldn't it?

Steve: More likely a penalty shot.

Karen: Rinse the beets well, cut them into four pieces, and steam them for 15 minutes or until they are soft enough to puncture with a fork. Now you'll have to peel them and do remember to cover your hands.

Steve: Now, how do you serve them up?

Karen: I like to toss beets with balsamic vinaigrette, feta or goat cheese, and some basil, or simply toss them in a salad. You can make a great appetizer by chopping beets into small pieces and dressing them with olive oil, balsamic vinegar, or a dressing of your choice. While you're at it, toss in that goat cheese, then scoop the mixture into endive leaves.

Steve: What the heck are endives? I don't think I've heard you mention those before.

Karen: A woman has to hold a few things back. Endives are a leaf vegetable that belongs to the daisy family. They're great for salads. Now, if all this sounds like too much work, or you're in a hurry, you can buy cooked and peeled beets. It doesn't get any easier that that.

Steve: Caveman style?

Karen: Yes, you can eat beets raw, but you will want to peel them first, then grate them into dishes like coleslaw or on top of a salad. Now here's something you may not know. You can also eat the beet leaves. They're called beet greens and they are similar to Swiss chard and spinach in the texture.

Steve: I'm guessing they're loaded with vitamins.

Karen: They're an excellent source of vitamins A and C, both of which are powerful antioxidants that help protect us at a cellular level. This is a great food to include in your diet to protect your vision. It's loaded with lutein. Also, 1 cup of beet greens contains over 800% of your daily requirement for vitamin K, which plays an important role in bone health. It helps to maintain bone mass by securing calcium molecules inside the bones.

Steve: Once you cut the greens from the root, how do you store them?

Karen: Put them in an air-tight container for up to 4 days. You'll know they're starting to turn bad if the leaves become yellow or wilted. Okay, go ahead and say it.

Steve: How do you cook them?

Karen: One of the easiest ways to prepare beet greens is to simply boil them. Once rinsed, you will want to layer the leaves and then cut them into strips. Toss them in boiling water for only 1 minute. The greens should remain deep green in color and should not be mushy.

Steve: Yep. No one likes mushy beet greens, especially if you've never had them. Okay, bottom line, guys. Beets and beet greens are loaded with vitamins, antioxidants, and other things to make you Superman. We can't guarantee you'll fly, but you'll certainly look better in tights! And if you find yourself in the produce section of your grocery store, remember to use the AC/DC line with the produce manager. Tell him you're looking for dirty beets, done dirt cheap. You'll make his day, especially if you bring your guitar and amp in the cart.

Bok Choy – Delicious and Cool Sounding

Steve: One of my favorite vegetables just happens to be one of the healthiest in the entire universe.

Karen: Are you sure you can make that claim?

Steve: What do you mean?

Karen: It's a big universe out there and you haven't exactly visited every corner of the galaxy.

Steve: You don't know that.

Karen: Interesting.

Steve: Before I married a nutritionist, I thought bok choy was something you yelled out in martial arts class. Booooooooook choy! Boy, was I wrong.

Karen: Yes, you were. Bok choy, commonly known as Chinese cabbage, has been cultivated for over six thousand years.

Steve: Thus the martial arts tie-in to the story.

Karen: Totally missed that.

Steve: Perhaps if you were as well traveled as I …

Karen: Right. This vegetable, bok choy, is in the same family as broccoli, cabbage, cauliflower, and Brussels sprouts.

Steve: And bok choy is great for salads and soups, and it can be sautéed in a pan the way we do at home. Aside from tasting great, bok choy has some terrific health benefits which Karen will now tell you about.

Karen: No, you can go ahead. You know the health benefits, unless you haven't been listening to me.

Steve: Me not listen to you? You're kidding, right? Guys always listen to their wives. We may not always look like we are, but we are, even when we're watching football.

Karen: Okay, then tell them about the health benefits of bok choy.

Steve: Okay, maybe I will.

Karen: Waiting.

Steve: I'm just ramping up. Okay, here we go. Bok choy is a rich source of many essential vitamins such as vitamin A, which supports your immune system, improves vision, and makes your teeth and bones amazingly strong. It also provides vitamin C, which is loaded with free-radical blasting antioxidants.

Karen: I'm impressed.

Steve: How about this? It's also packed with folate, which lowers your risk of heart disease, and B6 which helps with the formation of red blood cells and antibodies.

Karen: I commend you. You certainly know your bok choy vitamins.

Steve: Like I said, bok choy is one of my favorites. Unless, of course, you weren't listening.

Karen: What do you mean? Of course I was listening. Women always listen to their husbands. We may not always look like we are, but we are, even if we're busy keeping the world running.

Steve: As opposed to running the world?

Karen: You got it. By the way, you forgot to mention that bok choy is loaded with beta-carotene.

Steve: Yes, an antioxidant believed to reduce the risk of many Cancers.

Karen: How about calcium and potassium?

Steve: I'm getting there. Jeez. It's like you're amped up on green tea, or something.

Karen: Sorry. Your excitement for bok choy is infectious.

Steve: Yes it is. Bok choy is amazingly cheap to buy at the store.

Karen: Ding. Ding. Ding.

Steve: Yes, we have a winner. At the farmer's market this morning, we picked up three heads of bok choy for a buck! To see a short video on how simple it is to cook, visit our YouTube Channel at Youtube.com/NutritionalChoice.

Karen: Bottom line, gentlemen. Bok choy, as Steve says, rocks! Amazingly healthy, quick and easy to cook, inexpensive, delicious, and cool sounding when you say to the produce manager, "Excuse me, where be the bok choy?"

Steve: Nice!

Karen: One last tip. Baby bok choy has less nutrients than matured bok choy.

Steve: So look for the bok choy that's out of diapers and wearing big boy pants.

Karen: Oh brother. Another advantage of mature bok choy is that it's cheaper!

Steve: Score!

Cancer-Busting Broccoli Sprouts

Karen: In 1992, researchers from Johns Hopkins University identified a highly concentrated phytochemical, sulforaphane, found in broccoli and broccoli sprouts. It is believed to reduce the risk of developing Cancer by boosting the liver's detoxification enzymes, which in turn sweep away Cancer-causing chemicals that have accumulated in the body.

Steve: I'm big on phytochemicals.

Karen: Oh really?

Steve: Did I tell you I once knew a dog name Fido-chemical.

Karen: And did you also know a dog named Detoxification Enzymes?

Steve: No, just Detox. He peed like a fire hose and pooped like a Play-Doh machine.

Karen: Okay, I'm going to try to erase that image from my mind by talking about broccoli. Broccoli and broccoli sprouts are also beneficial to our digestive tracts and protect against Stomach Cancer. It's the sulforaphane compound that destroys the H. pylori bacteria responsible for peptic ulcers.

Steve: As good as broccoli is for you, a lot of people don't care for it or the after effects for some.

Karen: Go ahead and say it. I know you want to.

Steve: I have no idea what you're talking about. Oh, you mean farting?

Karen: I knew you couldn't help yourself.

Steve: And neither can a lot of people who eat broccoli in public. You either got to hold it in or start crop dusting.

Karen: Crop dusting?

Steve: Silently passing gas while walking through a crowd.

Not that I've ever done that, but I have been a victim of someone's unsettled lunch.

Karen: Let's move on to broccoli sprouts.

Steve: Yes, let's do.

Karen: Broccoli sprouts, which look like other types of sprouts you might put on a salad or sandwich, contain 20 to 50-times more of the Cancer-protecting compound than whole broccoli. To put that in perspective, you would get the same amount in half-cup of sprouts as you would in one-and-a-quarter pound of cooked broccoli.

Steve: And you could easily put a half-cup of sprouts on a salad.

Karen: Exactly.

Steve: And for those that don't like broccoli, the good news is the sprouts don't taste like broccoli. They have a peppery flavor. In addition to salads, you can use them on sandwiches, wraps, pita pockets, tacos, burritos, stir in with a bowl of soup, or mix them in with rice pilaf.

Karen: You can purchase broccoli sprouts at most grocery stores, and they can be stored in the refrigerator for about 2 weeks, depending on how long they were on the shelf.

Steve: But we don't do that, do we, my nutritionist?

Karen: No, we don't, my man who likes to talk about crop dusting. We like to grow our own. It takes about 4-6 days to grow broccoli sprouts in your kitchen, using a sprouter and seeds. The reason why I like to grow my own is it's not only a lot cheaper, it's also fun to watch it grow.

Steve: Just like a Chia Pet.

Karen: And when you grow them at home, you know they're clean and free of bacteria. You can buy sprouters in most kitchen-supply stores, or if you have a mason jar, you can just buy a sprouting lid with tiny holes so you can rinse and drain the seeds.

Steve: The seeds are a little harder to find, though.

Karen: They can be, but I suggest you check your local health food stores – the smaller ones tend to carry them but the larger markets generally don't.

Steve: Bottom line, guys. If you're gonna crop dust…

Karen: Wrong bottom.

Steve: Bottom line, guys. Broccoli is an amazing food for you, and even more amazing are broccoli sprouts. Whether they're store bought, or home grown, we're talking some serious Cancer prevention as well as other health benefits.

Karen: That should do it.

Steve: I'm going to go rinse our sprouts.

Karen: And I'm going to rinse my hands. I've been petting Riley and man does he need a bath!

Eggplant – Nature's Purple Football

Steve: We all know that fruits and vegetables are good for us, but most of us don't eat a variety of them. That's why we want to talk to you about eggplant.

Karen: A lot of people are intimidated by this vegetable.

Steve: I know I am. Freaky little alien pod.

Karen: They're not freaky, they're delicious. Many people are just unsure how to pick out a ripe eggplant and what to do with it once they get it home.

Steve: I like to poke it with a stick to make sure it's not alive.

Karen: You do not.

Steve: You're right. We have a beagle, and if anything were about to hatch out of it, like a stranger from another planet, our dog would be all over it.

Karen: Before we talk about how to pick out an eggplant and how to cook it, let's first talk about the health benefits of this wonderful vegetable.

Steve: Let's.

Karen: Eggplant contains nasunin, a potent antioxidant that protects cell membranes from damage. Studies have shown that it protects the lipids or fat of our brain cell membranes, which shields us from free radicals that can alter how our cells communicate with messenger molecules. It's that same phytonutrient that gives eggplant its purple color so you need to eat the skin to get the most benefit.

Steve: Yep. I've seen the movie.

Karen: What movie?

Steve: *The Color Purple.*

Karen: I walked right into that.

Steve: Yes, you did.

Karen: Eggplant may also help you sleep better since it contains tryptophan.

Steve: That's a snoozer.

Karen: Eggplant contains many heart healthy nutrients, such as fiber, folate, vitamins B-3 and B-6, along with magnesium and potassium. Other healthy phytochemicals in eggplant have been studied for their effect on lowering cholesterol.

Steve: And the results were? Drum roll please …

Karen: Animal studies have shown that when eggplant juice was consumed, blood cholesterol was lowered and blood flow improved, due to the walls of the blood vessels relaxing.

Steve: And as an added bonus, 1 cup of cooked eggplant is only 28 calories.

Karen: That's right. Now, when choosing an eggplant, you want to look for one that is firm and feels heavy for its size.

Steve: Reminds me of a girl I once dated in high school.

Karen: I'll ignore that. You can tell if an eggplant is ripe by gently pressing on the skin. If it bounces back, it's ripe. The skin should be smooth and shiny.

Steve: Just like the air-brushed models in *Maxim* magazine.

Karen: Oh, so now you admit they're air-brushed.

Steve: Yes, and if you gently press on their skin and it bounces back, they're ready to date.

Karen: If the eggplant isn't organic, it's best to peel it because conventionally grown eggplant will be coated with wax and that wax can trap in pesticides. Try to purchase organic eggplant so you can eat the skin. No comments?

Steve: I don't know what you mean.

Karen: I just assumed you were going to interject a cannibalism joke when I mentioned eating the skin.

Steve: Cannibalism isn't something you joke about.

Karen: I agree.

Steve: That's why cannibals don't eat comedians. They taste funny.

Karen: Eggplant tends to have a bitter taste, but if properly prepared that can be avoided. Simply cut off the ends of the eggplant and slice it into half-inch pieces. Sprinkle the slices with sea salt, cover with a towel, and let sit for 1 hour. This pulls out the water and reduces bitterness.

Steve: You can add chopped eggplant to your stir-fries.

Karen: That's a delicious way to eat eggplant.

Steve: How about an eggplant sandwich? I had one of those not too long ago. You simply sauté sliced eggplant until brown on both sides and top with tomato, cheese, and onion.

Karen: The next time you're in a Greek restaurant, try the moussaka. It's a great alternative to lasagna, with eggplant replacing the noodles.

Steve: Now, as I recall, there are some people who should avoid eating eggplant.

Karen: Yes, and that's what I was going to say next.

Steve: Just keeping the conversation moving along.

Karen: People who should avoid eggplant are those who are prone to kidney stones, since eggplant contains a high level of oxalates. Likewise, if you suffer from Arthritis, know that eggplant is part of the nightshade family, and some people notice improvement in their symptoms when they avoid the nightshade vegetables, which also include potatoes, tomatoes, and sweet and hot peppers.

Steve: Ready for bottom line?

Karen: Maybe I should say it because you don't seem very confident about it.

Steve: What do you mean?

Karen: Well, if you were confident about your bottom line, you wouldn't have asked me if I was ready for it. You would have jumped right in and said it ... confidently.

Steve: All right. **Bottom line, guys. Despite looking like a purple alien football, eggplant is worth working into your diet because it has tremendous health benefits. Lots of heart healthy nutrients, and remember to buy it organic so you can eat the skin like a cannibal.**

Karen: I think we're done here.

Steve: I agree.

Karen: Hey! There's that confidence!

Take a Leek

Steve: Yep, nothing feels better than taking a big leek … from the produce section and putting it in your shopping cart.

Karen: You just love the name of this vegetable, don't you?

Steve: Oh, absolutely. What guy wouldn't?

Karen: I'm sure there are a few out there.

Steve: Poor saps. They're out of touch with their inner caveman child and not appreciating one of the national emblems of Wales. Leeks.

Karen: You just couldn't wait to get that out, could you?

Steve: Since lunch.

Karen: I hope it was worth it.

Steve: Oh, it was.

Karen: One of the earliest spring vegetables you will start to see at the farmer's market is leeks. They are in the same family as onions and garlic, just milder in flavor.

Steve: So if you tend to shy away from onions and garlic due to the smell or strong flavor, leeks are just the vegetable for you. Their mild onion-like taste means they can be used in place of onions or scallions.

Karen: I wish you would start eating sliced leeks on your sandwiches.

Steve: What? You don't like onion breath?

Karen: Does anyone like onion breath?

Steve: Our beagle does.

Karen: You can sleep with the beagle.

Steve: On second thought, maybe I'll try leeks instead of raw onions.

Karen: Good choice. Leeks have many of the same benefits that you find in garlic and onion, such as the allicin. This is a sulphur compound that can boost your immune system. This sulphur compound is beneficial to maintaining normal blood-sugar levels and acts as an antibacterial and antiviral agent.

Steve: Okay, now let's talk some dirt. The key to leeks is getting them dirt-free. You take a sharp knife, chop off the bottom root end, and do the same with the dark green tops. This leaves you with the white and light green parts. Rinse the leeks. Cut them in half length-wise and spread out the pieces. Now this is when you want to rinse them really good because the dirt likes to hide.

Karen: You make it sound like dirt is a living thing.

Steve: How so?

Karen: You said, "The dirt likes to hide."

Steve: Yes, it does.

Karen: Dirt can't "like" to hide. Rather, dirt can be hidden.

Steve: Which is why I recommend thoroughly washing it. Next, you slice the pieces of leeks into thin strips.

Karen: Leeks are great on top of salads. You can also lightly sauté them, or top them with fresh Parmesan cheese and serve this as a side dish. The most popular dish using leeks is, of course, potato leek soup. You'll find a yummy recipe for potato leek soup in the Recipes section of my website.

Steve: Yummy?

Karen: It is.

Steve: I agree, but I'm not so sure "yummy" is the best word to use for our guy readers.

Karen: Okay, do-over. Visit the Recipes section of my website for a delicious soup recipe using Leeks. Better?

Steve: A little bit. Try again. Tougher this time.

Karen: Visit the Recipes section of my website for a bad-ass, rockin' potato leek soup recipe that you can eat out of a hubcap!

Steve: You nailed it!

Karen: Bottom line, gentlemen. If you don't take kindly to onions or scallions, try leeks. They can boost your immune system, help maintain normal blood sugar levels, and have antibacterial and antiviral properties. Leeks are not as strong tasting as most onions but they sure do look like amped-up, testosterone-charged scallions.

Steve: Oh yeah!

Karen: And remember … they're at their freshest in the early spring when the butterflies are out and the flowers begin to bloom.

Steve: Ah jeez.

Hold the Pasta – Go Spaghetti Squash

Karen: Now here's a vegetable that all guys should like.

Steve: Why is that?

Karen: Unlike your description of an eggplant as a football, a spaghetti squash really looks like a football.

Steve: Sort of. More like a yellow rugby ball.

Karen: I don't know what a rugby ball looks like.

Steve: It looks like a spaghetti squash, but for your sake, we'll stick with football. Now, guys, a word of warning. Don't be tempted to throw your spaghetti squash to your wife unless she's a good catch! An eggplant is good for a down and out pattern in the kitchen because it's soft. However, the spaghetti squash could cost you a nose job and a year sleeping on the couch!

Karen: Spaghetti squash is delicious, really easy to cook, and above all … very healthy.

Steve: The best way to cook a spaghetti squash is to steam it. First, take a heavy sharp knife and cut the spaghetti squash in half length-wise. It's not an easy cut so if you feel uneasy about it, have them slice it in half at the store. Next, you scoop out all the seeds and gook in the middle.

Karen: There's no gook.

Steve: Okay, slimy strands and seeds. Don't worry about wearing gloves, it's not going to hurt you. Once the middle is cleaned out, place one or both halves in a steamer with the cut side facing down. Our steamer takes roughly 30 minutes to cook both halves. Another option is to use a big pot with boiling water and a steamer insert.

Karen: Test the squash to make sure it's done. You do this by scraping the center of the squash with a fork. If it comes out easily in noodle-like strands, it's done.

Steve: Most every guy I know loves traditional spaghetti and meat sauce. With this recipe, you're simply replacing the pasta with spaghetti squash and adding healthy sauce and organic meat. Why organic meat? If you knew what was inside most regular ground beef, you wouldn't be asking such a question. Trust me. Go organic and grass-fed. It's better for you, no hormones, no added water. Just good meat.

Karen: Coming up is our recipe for making a truly delicious meat sauce to go over your spaghetti squash.

Steve: If you don't like to read, or can't read ... which is highly unlikely since you're reading this book, unless of course you're just looking at the pictures ... you can also watch our spaghetti squash video on our YouTube channel at Youtube.com\NutritionalChoice.

Karen: Go ahead, Steve, and give yourself credit for shooting and editing it. You did a good job with our home camera.

Steve: It's not quite the Food Channel but it came out pretty good if I don't say so myself.

Karen: As a backup, here's the written recipe. The ingredients are:

- 1 spaghetti squash about the size of a Nerf football.
- 1 jar organic spaghetti sauce with no added sugar.
- 1 pound organic ground beef ... grass-fed if you can get it.

Steve: And here are the directions:

- Wash the outside of the spaghetti squash – some worm may have slobbered on it!
- *Carefully* cut the spaghetti squash in half with a sturdy butcher knife. (Don't attempt Samurai style unless you're certified crazy.)
- Scoop out the middle (seeds and surrounding moist strands) with a spoon. (Flashbacks of Halloween)

- Steam both halves of the spaghetti squash cut-side-down for about 20-30 minutes. (It's done when you can push a fork into it and retrieve strands, and the strands are a bit crunchy.)
- While the squash is steaming, brown the ground beef in a frying pan.
- Heat the spaghetti sauce in a pan and add the browned meat.
- When the spaghetti squash is done, take a fork and scrape out the insides into a bowl.
- Dish out some spaghetti squash on plates and cover it with the meat sauce.
- We like to add crushed red pepper and fresh grated Parmesan cheese (optional).

Karen: Bottom line, gentlemen …

Steve: Wait! It's my turn. Remember the gentlemen overload thing? **Bottom line, guys. Spaghetti squash is low-carb, low-calorie, easy to make, and healthy. Plus you get to use a big knife to cut the spaghetti squash in half! Just watch your fingers and other body parts. If you're secure enough with your manhood, take the easy way out and ask the produce guy to do it. He'll appreciate the break in routine from stacking zucchinis and shucking corn, and most likely he'll be able to catch your "Hail Mary" pass as you throw a perfect spiral.**

Sweet Potato Home Alabama

Karen: Sweet potatoes make an ideal replacement for white potatoes. They have fewer calories, more fiber, and a lot more flavor.

Steve: And we know what fiber does.

Karen: Keeps you regular?

Steve: Oh, much more than that, my nutritionist-wife. Insoluble fiber is like a sponge. It sucks up water and toxins, and it promotes efficient elimination by helping you create a really bulky stool.

Karen: Wow. That was quite impressive.

Steve: Yeah, you know guys. We like bulky stools. Makes us feel productive.

Karen: No. Actually I didn't know that but thanks for that information … I think.

Steve: Insoluble fiber is great for relieving constipation. Additionally, fiber from vegetables, fruits, and their skins, along with the hulls of whole grains, can relieve constipation.

Karen: If you drink enough fluids. Otherwise, it could plug you up.

Steve: Precisely!

Karen: How about we transition back to sweet potatoes?

Steve: Transition away.

Karen: Sweet potatoes are an excellent source of beta-carotene, and a very good source of vitamin C. These nutrients can be helpful in reducing inflammation. Some recent animal studies have shown that sweet potatoes help stabilize blood sugar levels thanks to the beta-carotene.

Steve: Okay, let's jump over to shopping. What do you look for when buying sweet potatoes, other than one of those hard to open little plastic bags?

Karen: You want to avoid sweet potatoes that are in the refrigerated section of the store. And do not refrigerate them when you get them home. The moisture can alter the taste and cause them to sprout.

Steve: Takes me back to third grade science class with the sweet potato suspended in water with toothpicks.

Karen: Exactly. You also want to look for sweet potatoes that are firm without a lot of blemishes or cracks. They will keep for over a week in a cool dark space.

Steve: Next stop on the Nutrition Railroad. Preparation, minus the "H."

Karen: One of the easiest ways to prepare sweet potatoes is by steaming them. You can cut them up into cubes and steam them for 7-10 minutes depending on the size of your cubes. Top with some butter, real butter not margarine, and eat. You can also peel them before steaming, then mash them up with a drizzle of olive oil or butter and season with salt and pepper. Or try mixing in some cinnamon or sprinkle the mashed sweet potato with shredded coconut and chopped nuts for a sweet crunchy side dish.

Steve: You're making me hungry.

Karen: My personal favorite is to bake them. I start with organic sweet potatoes.

Steve: … So you can eat the skin. See? I've been listening.

Karen: You poke holes in the sweet potato, coat the potato with olive oil and sea salt, and then bake it at 400 degrees for 25-30 minutes. The olive oil and salt gives it such a nice flavor that you don't need to add anything. But you can add butter if you like.

Steve: No margarine.

Karen: Yes, no margarine.

Steve: Real organic butter.

Karen: Yes, real organic butter.

Steve: From real cows.

Karen: Hormone-free, grass-fed cows.

Steve: I think we've covered sweet potatoes.

Karen: Yes, I believe we have. **Bottom line, gentlemen. Incorporate sweet potatoes into your diet. They're not only good for you with lots of beta-carotene, vitamin C, and other nutrients, they're much more tasty than regular potatoes and they're amazing on the grill.**

Steve: Good job incorporating the grill. Guys like that.

Karen: That's what I figured.

Steve: Tailgate grilling?

Karen: Sure. Throw in a couple of cold brewskis, grilled sweet potatoes, and you'll have the Bud Girls swarming your rig faster than you can say anti-inflammatory.

Steve: Nice!

Karen: I thought you'd like that.

Steve: Indeed.

For a boatload of healthy product suggestions, visit:
IMarriedaNutritionist.com
Click on "Karen's Selections."

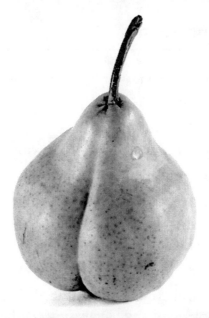

THE FRUIT STUFF

CHAPTER 4

*"Why not go out on a limb? That's where the fruit is." ~ **Will Rogers***

*"I'm thinking Will Rogers may have over-estimated how much a limb can hold, especially if you're fat." ~ **Steve Roth***

Avocado – Odacova Spelled Backwards

Karen: Avocados are truly a wonderful food.

Steve: Unfortunately, many people steer clear of them because of their high-fat value.

Karen: Yes, but two-thirds of that fat is monounsaturated and good for the heart. If anyone has followed a Mediterranean diet, they know it emphasizes monounsaturated fats like avocado and olive oil.

Steve: I once saw a calendar of Mediterranean women all oiled up. Any correlation?

Karen: I don't think so.

Steve: One was peeling an avocado … with her teeth.

Karen: Still no correlation.

Steve: Another was eating an avocado while smiling.

Karen: As long as she was ingesting the avocado, yes, there may be a correlation.

Steve: I knew it!

Karen: Avocados have many health benefits, including lowering LDL cholesterol and increasing the health-promoting HDL cholesterol. They're high in potassium, which supports blood-pressure regulation, and avocados are a good source of fiber, folic acid, and vitamin B6 … all essential nutrients for a healthy heart.

Steve: Pass the guacamole. And let me flip back to that Bloody Mary recipe.

Karen: That would be good right now, wouldn't it?

Steve: Oh, absolutely. We need to plant an avocado tree. I'll go dig a hole.

Karen: A 2005 study published in the *Journal of Nutrition* found that by adding avocados to salads, there is an increased absorption of the health-promoting phytonutrients from the vegetables.

Steve: I wonder how big a hole I'll need to dig.

Karen: Let's stay focused. You can dig later … with the dog.

Steve: Good idea. He's a four-legged bulldozer.

Karen: Now you never want to eat an over-ripened avocado, you know the ones that have separated from the pit or have brown spots or dark streaks. These brown markings are a sign of free radical formation, which is what we want to avoid as much as possible.

Steve: Explain free radicals.

Karen: Well, imagine free radicals as rust spreading over your car.

Steve: Okay, good analogy. I'm sure these guys can relate.

Karen: The more free radicals you have, the more damage they will do to your body.

Steve: Sorry to say, guys, but we're rusting away. You know, I'm thinking they should change the name of that to imprisoned radicals. "Free" sounds too positive and uplifting.

Karen: Now I'm sure you've cut into an over-ripe avocado and thought, hey, no problem, I can eat around the brown spot. Trust me, it's not worth it!

Steve: Yeah, who wants to deal with imprisoned free radicals? Oh, yeah, that sounds so much better.

Karen: Avocados are great in salads and wraps. I mash half an avocado and spread it on my sandwiches instead of mayonnaise. And chunks of avocado taste wonderful in salsa.

Steve: Me? I eat half of an avocado for breakfast with a hard-boiled egg and cottage cheese. Lots of healthy fat to start off the day.

Karen: It's an easy breakfast that is so good for you.

Steve: Bottom line, guys. You don't have to wait for the next big game to eat avocados in guacamole. Make avocados a regular part of your diet. You'll get lots of health benefits including lowering your LDL and kicking up your good HDL cholesterol.

Karen: Imprisoned radicals? You're so goofy sometimes.

Steve: That's what Minnie Mouse said.

Blueberries Keep the Blues Away

Karen: As we age, many of us will see a decline in mental capabilities, whether it's memory loss, trouble thinking of the right word, or being forgetful.

Steve: What were you just saying?

Karen: That's not memory loss, that's just not listening. We often blame memory problems on getting old, when in fact the two major causes of mental decline are oxidative damage and inflammation. Conditions that can be prevented!

Steve: That's good news.

Karen: You bet it is. The National Institute of Aging conducted a study with rats on how blueberries may protect the brain. The two groups were both given a toxic chemical that causes the same kind of damage to the brain as we see in Alzheimer's. The outcome was that the rats that had a diet rich in blueberries, prior to having been exposed to the chemical, showed much less decline. That's powerful protection!

Steve: I'm liking what I'm hearing. Blueberries are delicious.

Karen: This is significant research when you consider that one in eight people over the age of sixty-five have Alzheimer's.

Steve: That's a scary number.

Karen: Blueberries contain almost 40% more of the same antioxidant found in red wine.

Steve: So I should have a glass of blueberries after work?

Karen: It's this antioxidant, resveratrol, that protects the brain from oxidative stress.

Steve: Which is …?

Karen: Oxidative stress is what happens when the cells of the body die off due to a lack of antioxidants such as resveratrol. Think of a car that's rusting … eventually the metal will crumble. That is what oxidative stress does to our "frames."

Steve: Great analogy.

Karen: Blueberries are in peak season from May through October. Get them while they're in season, stock up, and freeze them for the winter time.

Steve: Some simple ways I incorporate the powerful antioxidants of blueberries into my diet is by including them in smoothies, throwing a handful into my bowl of oatmeal, mixing them in with my yogurt, and even tossing fresh blueberries into salads.

Karen: And remember, organic is preferable when it comes to blueberries. They are number three on the "Dirty Dozen" list of the most heavily sprayed crops. Personally, I don't buy them unless they're organic.

Steve: And I don't eat them unless they're organic, mainly because you buy them.

Karen: So when I find them at a good price, I stock up and freeze them. **Bottom line, gentlemen. Blueberries are a powerful tool in your arsenal for maintaining good health. Antioxidants up the yin-yang. So simple to incorporate into your diet. So delicious.**

Steve: Up the yin-yang?

Karen: Problem?

Steve: I've just never heard it called that before?

Karen: What?

Steve: Well, you know …

Karen: It's not that. Yin-yang is the belief in the value of balance.

Steve: I knew that.

Karen: Never doubted it for one moment.

Steve: I was just testing you. You passed … up the yin-yang.

If You Cantaloupe, May as Well Have a Wedding

Karen: Ready to roll into this next fruit?

Steve: Oh, I get it because a cantaloupe is round and it rolls.

Karen: No. Actually because your chair is on rollers and you're way across the room scratching the dog. I need you to roll over here.

Steve: Rollin', rollin', rollin', keep those wheels moving, desk chair!

Karen: Cantaloupe is an excellent source of vitamins A and C, two powerful antioxidants that can prevent and repair damage done by free radicals.

Steve: You heard about free radicals two fruits back, so we're not going to regurgitate the imprisoned radical thing. Just remember, free radicals can lead to disease and cause our bodies to age.

Karen: In addition to vitamins A and C, cantaloupe contains a good amount of beta-carotene. In fact, it's the beta-carotene that gives cantaloupe its rich orange color.

Steve: I didn't know that.

Karen: Life is just full of surprises. It's also beta-carotene that promotes healthy vision and may prevent cataracts.

Steve: Cantaloupe is also a heart healthy food!

Karen: Why are you looking at me?

Steve: Because I'm teeing up the subject so you can drive it down the fairway with nutrition expertise.

Karen: Well, you can do some of the driving, too.

Steve: Yes, but you do it so much better. Really, you do.

Karen: Cantaloupe is a very good source of potassium, which helps maintain healthy blood pressure. It's also a good source of both folate and vitamin B6, which breaks down homocysteine in the blood. Homocysteine is an amino acid in the blood that when elevated can lead to stroke and heart disease.

Steve: I'm eating more cantaloupe starting tomorrow.

Karen: Terrific. Here's how you pick one out at the store.

Steve: But you generally buy the cantaloupe.

Karen: Yes, but there may be a time when you need to buy the cantaloupe.

Steve: Such as?

Karen: When you're at the store buying beer for the Superbowl and I call you on your cell and say, "We need some cantaloupe."

Steve: Hasn't happened.

Karen: Could.

Steve: Probably not.

Karen: Maybe so. You never know.

Steve: Okay, you wore me down. Say, hypothetically, I were to purchase cantaloupe. What should I look for?

Karen: The first thing you do when picking out a cantaloupe is smell the small circle where the stem came off. It should have a sweet aroma, and it should feel heavy for its size.

Steve: Don't worry. I won't repeat the joke about the girl in high school feeling heavy for her size. And, no, I didn't smell her when I picked her up to see if she had a sweet aroma.

Karen: Glad to hear that. Now assuming you buy a ripe cantaloupe, it should last about 5 days.

Steve: If plain old sliced cantaloupe is too boring for you, try using half a cantaloupe as a bowl and fill it up with cottage cheese and sprinkle with pumpkin seeds. Or go crazy and fill the half cantaloupe with Greek yogurt and top with chopped nuts.

Karen: Outstanding!

Steve: I may be lazy when it comes to buying cantaloupe, but I do watch you work in the kitchen, especially when I'm hungry.

Karen: So does the dog.

Steve: Yeah, but I can see much better from my angle. He's on the floor looking up.

Karen: I like to prepare a delicious fruit salad by taking chunks of cantaloupe and squeezing some lemon or lime juice over it. I then toss it with goat cheese and balsamic vinegar.

Steve: And on hot days, whip up some cantaloupe in a blender and freeze it. I know it sounds a little strange but it comes out like sorbet. To sweeten it up, add some xylitol.

Karen: This is a great fruit to add to your diet because its nutrients support heart health and healthy vision. It's delicious and low in calories at 56 calories for a cup of cubed cantaloupe.

Steve: Bottom line, Dudes …

Karen: Dudes? What happened to "Guys"?

Steve: Thought I would mix it up a little. **Bottom line, Dudes, cantaloupe is great for your health with lots of vitamins A and C to keep your frame rust-free and beta-carotene for healthy peepers. Plus, cantaloupes are fun to roll around in the kitchen like lawn bowling, and most of all they're orange.**

Karen: What's so important about orange?

Steve: The Home Depot.

Karen: Got it. A visual tie-in. Guys are so predictable some-times.

Steve: On behalf of every guy in the world … thank you.

Grapefruit – Bigger than a Grape but Still a Fruit

Steve: When I think of grapefruit, it takes me back to my early years on this planet.

Karen: As opposed to time spent on other planets?

Steve: Figure of speech.

Karen: Just providing clarification for our readers. I don't want them to think you were a space traveler.

Steve: Glad you didn't say space cadet.

Karen: I would never call you that.

Steve: Thank you.

Karen: Because I know for certain you never went to space academy.

Steve: As I was saying … grapefruit reminds me of my growing up years. My father, who was quite the planner, used to not only set the table for breakfast the night before, he would painstakingly prepare grapefruit for the morning meal.

Karen: It was part of his daily routine.

Steve: Yes it was. He would cut the grapefruit in half, and then with a special curved knife he would cut around each piece so it could easily come out with a spoon.

Karen: That's some serious prep work.

Steve: At the breakfast table, we would sprinkle a little sugar on top of the grapefruit, and when all the fruit was eaten, we would put the grapefruit skin in the palm of our hands and squeeze the remaining juice onto the spoon, and then down the hatch it went.

Karen: Great story! When grapefruit is in peak season, winter through early spring, it has the highest concentration of nutrients, the most flavor, and lowest cost.

Steve: And if your neighbor has a tree that hangs over your fence, that's the best deal of all!

Karen: Let's talk about the health benefits of grapefruit.

Steve: Why are you looking at me?

Karen: I'm teeing it up.

Steve: Oh, okay. Grapefruit is a good source of fiber and contains pectin, a form of soluble fiber that traps fats.

Karen: Grapefruit pectin has been found to inhibit the build-up of fatty deposits on artery walls. Other heart-healthy components in grapefruit include potassium, which regulates blood pressure, lycopene in red and pink grapefruit which has been found to inhibit free radical damage of LDL cholesterol, and that white coat that is under the grapefruit skin contains flavonoids that may help lower LDL cholesterol.

Steve: I don't know about that white undercoating. Pretty bitter.

Karen: But some people do like the taste.

Steve: Guess that's what makes the grapefruit go round. Grapefruit is also an excellent source of vitamins C and A, which are very supportive for the immune system. And as timing would have it, grapefruit season coincides with winter flu season. Yes, the world works in mysterious ways.

Karen: Animal studies have shown that grapefruit and its isolated active compounds promote the death of Cancer cells while increasing the production of normal colon cells. And in human studies where subjects drank three six-ounce servings of grapefruit juice daily, it was found to reduce enzyme activity that activates Cancer-causing chemicals found in tobacco smoke.

Steve: Holy smokes!

Karen: Cigarettes? Not so holy.

Steve: Agree big time.

Karen: Grapefruit is also very low in calories at only 74 calories for a whole grapefruit!

Steve: Okay, guys, consider this. Say you're shopping solo at the grocery store, maybe buying beer for the big game. Your cell phone rings and you answer it. It's your wife or maybe girlfriend or even a sexy voice wrong number woman asking you to pick up some grapefruit while you're shopping.

Karen: A sexy voice wrong number asking you to buy grapefruit?

Steve: Just roll with it, okay? The guy needs to buy grapefruit. Dudes, how are you to know which ones are ripe and have the best flavor?

Karen: Why not ask the sexy voice girl?

Steve: And look like we don't know what we're doing in the grapefruit arena? No chance.

Karen: Yes, I could see how that could be a deal breaker.

Steve: Exactly. So here's how you pick out a grapefruit. Look for one with smooth thin skin that feels kind of heavy, like a geisha girl with rocks in her pocket. It'll most likely be juicy.

Karen: The grapefruit or the geisha girl?

Steve: The grapefruit. Unless, of course, the geisha girl is wearing those sweat pants with "Juicy" written across the back.

Karen: In addition to smooth skin and feeling heavy, a ripe grapefruit feels firm and the skin should spring back when pressure is applied.

Steve: And it's important to remember that grapefruit doesn't ripen once picked, so you need to buy one that's already ripe.

Karen: When it comes to storing grapefruit, they'll last for up to five days on the counter and up to 10 days in the refrigerator.

Steve: I think this would be a good time to talk about how to work grapefruit into your diet.

Karen: Perfect. The most basic way is to peel the grapefruit and eat the slices. You can also prepare grapefruit the way Steve's father did, if you have a lot of time on your hands. Grapefruit is also great in salads, especially good with spinach, avocado, and shrimp. You can also chop grapefruit into small pieces and add it to chicken or tuna salad. If you like tropical salsas, try grapefruit mixed with chili peppers, cilantro, and chopped avocado. Amazing!

Steve: Been there, eaten that.

Karen: A word of caution if you're on medications. Check with your doctor to see if grapefruit or grapefruit juice will interfere with your meds. It's better to be safe than sorry.

Steve: Yeah, you never want to be sorry unless you have to.

Karen: Bottom line, gentlemen. Grapefruit is refreshing and very healthy for you. Lots of heart-healthy properties, free radical damage protection, may lower cholesterol, and it kicks up your immune system. If you're not eating it now, consider including it in your diet.

Steve: Well, we certainly squeezed all the juice out of that topic.

Karen: Yes. And you didn't even have to stay up and prepare it the night before!

Kiwi – A Taste from Down Under

Steve: All around the world New Zealanders are referred to as "Kiwis." One might think it could be offensive since kiwis are small round green fruit, but it's not.

Karen: Offensive as in people might assume that New Zealanders are short, round people wearing green clothing?

Steve: Yes, or covered with moss.

Karen: Interesting logic.

Steve: Kiwi is also the name of a flightless bird which is native to New Zealand. It's the national symbol.

Karen: You're quite the kiwi expert.

Steve: Well, I don't like to brag about it.

Karen: So I guess the next question is do kiwi birds eat kiwi fruit?

Steve: Well, they are omnivores with 80% of their diet being made up of insects. They also eat berries and fruit, which could include kiwis.

Karen: Interesting, in a strange sort of way.

Steve: Enough about birds, let's talk fruit. The majority of kiwi fruit in our supermarket is imported from, you guessed it, New Zealand. And when it's winter here, it's summer there and peak season for this amazing fruit.

Karen: Kiwis contain a lot of antioxidants and phytonutrients that protect our DNA and help fight free radical damage.

Steve: And at 46 calories on average, they're an excellent source of vitamin C.

Karen: Did you know that a kiwi contains more vitamin C than an orange?

Steve: No, I didn't know that.

Karen: And two kiwis have more potassium than one banana?

Steve: Didn't know that either. How about roughage? I'm guessing kiwis are loaded with fiber.

Karen: Absolutely. Kiwis protect the heart by naturally lowering high cholesterol levels due to their high fiber content. Here's an interesting note.

Steve: We'll be the ones to decide if it's interesting or not.

Karen: An Italian study of six and seven-year-olds found that the more kiwi and citrus the children ate, the less likely they were to have respiratory issues such as Asthma, wheezing, and shortness of breath.

Steve: That's interesting.

Karen: Told you. Kiwi fruit also helps regulate blood pressure with its good source of potassium and magnesium, and it can assist with controlling blood sugar and lower your risk of blood clots.

Steve: Let's see a banana do that.

Karen: Let's not get down on bananas. They have their own set of health benefits.

Steve: Said the monkey with his hands on his hips.

Karen: The skin of the kiwi is definitely edible and healthy for you. In fact, it's pretty common for people in New Zealand and other place in the world to eat the whole fruit, skin and all.

Steve: Doesn't the kiwi rank low on the pesticide list?

Karen: Yes. Kiwi is number eight on the Environmental Working Groups "Clean 15" list.

Steve: So eating the skin isn't so bad.

Karen: At that level, it's a trade-off of the health benefits of eating the skin versus the little bit of pesticides on the skin.

Steve: What about the "hairy skin" issue?

Karen: Like you when you don't shave?

Steve: Exactly … not. Kiwi skin? I peel it. The fuzz thing doesn't work for me.

Karen: Guess that's what makes the kiwi go round.

Steve: Gee, where have I heard something like that before? Oh, I know. I said it.

Karen: Stealing from the best.

Steve: Nice recovery.

Karen: We chop up kiwis and put them in green salads or make them part of a fruit salad. We also toss kiwi pieces in yogurt, and even blend them in a smoothie.

Steve: And believe it or not, the enzymes in kiwi act as a meat tenderizer, so you can rub one out on the meat before cooking.

Karen: Excuse me, but did you just say, "Rub one out?"

Steve: I don't know, did I?

Karen: I believe you did.

Steve: Well, I meant to say, "Rub one on."

Karen: Thank you. Jeez, you're turning this book into an R-rated read.

Steve: Slip of the tongue. Rub one out. Rub one on. Happens to politicians all the time.

Karen: You can toss uncooked kiwi pieces and pine nuts into side dishes made with rice or quinoa to add flavor.

Steve: Bottom line, guys. If you're not eating kiwis, give it a whirl. They're really tasty, loaded with antioxidants, phytonutrients, and vitamins among other healthy things. Plus, by eating them, you're supporting a really cool group of people down under there.

Karen: Under there?

Steve: Under where?

Karen: Gotcha.

Nice Pear!

Steve: Pears are one of my favorite fruits, and it's not just because it's fun to yell out "Nice Pear!" in the produce section at the grocery store. I really do like … pears.

Karen: I don't know how to respond to that.

Steve: Some people like their pears soft, like I do, while other people like their pears firm.

Karen: Duly noted. Let's move on.

Steve: I think I heard someone at the door. Did you hear the knockers?

Karen: Pears promote good digestive health because of the high amount of fiber they contain. As we mentioned earlier, fiber is important in your diet not only to prevent constipation, but because fiber is also instrumental in sweeping out Cancer-causing chemicals in the colon.

Steve: I remember you telling me that copper deficiency is also associated with Colon Cancer.

Karen: Yes it is, and pears are a good source of copper, which is an important mineral that fights off free radical damage that damages our cells.

Steve: And they taste better than a handful of pennies. Like the way I tied up the copper topic?

Karen: Good job. Now the good news is that there are so many varieties of pears, you'll pretty much find them in the store year-around.

Steve: When you shop for pears, you'll notice that they are all generally hard. That's because they are picked early since they perish so quickly. Pears will ripen at home in about 3 to 4 days. Five to 8 if you like them soft, like I do.

Karen: When it comes to organic versus non–organic, it's best to buy organic pears because they are number 16 on the Environmental Working Group's list of foods with the highest amount of pesticide residue. By buying organic pears, you'll be able to safely eat the skin which is a good source of dietary fiber.

Steve: And dietary fiber keeps Mr. Hankey, the Christmas Poo, right on schedule.

Karen: *South Park?* Really?

Steve: Don't get me started on the Mr. Hankey song.

Karen: You can slice pears and toss them into a green salad with blue cheese and red onion. One of my favorites!

Steve: Or try adding diced pears to chicken salad.

Karen: It's really delicious.

Steve: Or simply eat them as is. They're a convenient take-along snack.

Karen: Bottom line, gentlemen. Pears … THE FRUIT … are a great addition to your diet. Among other things, they're loaded with vitamin C, copper, fiber, and are low in calories.

Steve: Soft or hard, they're delicious.

Karen: We're done.

Pineapple – Peel It Danno!

Karen: Overindulging during a holiday meal, or any meal for that matter, can cause digestive upset.

Steve: I remember one Thanksgiving I ate so much I was full 6-hours afterwards.

Karen: I'm glad I wasn't around the next morning.

Steve: Till death do us fart.

Karen: The next time you overeat, try something different instead of reaching for an antacid, which may contain aluminum, and can lead to kidney stones and can block nutrient and mineral absorption ... Try eating some pineapple.

Steve: How come you've never mentioned this before?

Karen: I was waiting for you to take me to Hawaii.

Steve: Hawaii?

Karen: It would have been more appropriate to share this health tidbit while drinking Mai Tais on the beach at sunset.

Steve: Well, slap me with a grass skirt and call me a victim of poor vacation planning.

Karen: Pineapple contains an active enzyme called bromelain that functions as a digestive aid. The fruit must be eaten raw to get this benefit because cooked and canned pineapple contain no bromelain.

Steve: Yessiree. There's something very primitive about buying a whole pineapple in the store, taking it home, and whacking it open with the biggest knife in the drawer.

Karen: Must be a guy thing. I don't think I've ever heard a woman express a need like that.

Steve: *Kill Bill?*

Karen: Okay, maybe one.

Steve: So what's the deal with this bromelain that's in raw pineapple?

Karen: Bromelain is a protein-digesting enzyme. Eating a little pineapple 1 to 2 hours before or after a big meal can support healthy digestion.

Steve: I am so going to remember this.

Karen: Pineapple can also reduce inflammation. If you suffer from sore throats, Arthritis, respiratory conditions, or bad sinuses, try adding this fruit to your diet for its anti–inflammatory qualities. When using this as an anti–inflammatory, be sure to eat it on an empty stomach to get the full effect.

Steve: Done.

Karen: Pineapple is also an excellent source of vitamin C, which we know is a powerful antioxidant.

Steve: Pretty low in calories, too.

Karen: Absolutely. Around 75 calories for 1 cup.

Steve: If you're intimidated about purchasing a pineapple because you're not quite sure how to pick out a good one, all you need to know is that a pineapple should have a sweet aroma and feel heavy for its size.

Karen: Like George Clooney with rocks in his pocket.

Steve: Good one, but how do you know George Clooney smells good?

Karen: A woman knows these things.

Steve: Okay, back to the ripe pineapple thing. You'll know a pineapple is ripe if you slightly press on the skin and it bounces back.

Karen: Yes, and like grapefruit, pineapple doesn't ripen after it's picked. So be sure to buy a ripe one.

Steve: Yeah. The last thing you want to be stuck with is holding a hard one.

Karen: Ignoring that.

Steve: Okay. Suit yourself, but non-ripe pineapples are nothing to ignore.

Karen: Moving on ... I recommend eating raw pineapple whenever possible. One of the best ways to do that is by adding pineapple to a fruit salad containing kiwi, mango, and papaya.

Steve: You're making me hungry again.

Karen: Other ways you can incorporate this healthy fruit into your diet include adding pineapple to marinades to help tenderize the meat. Try adding pineapple to fruit smoothies or salads, including chicken salad.

Steve: Anything else?

Karen: As a matter of fact, yes. For those who are sensitive to tomato-based foods, try making a tropical salsa which is delicious on baked fish and pork.

Steve: Think we should share your recipe?

Karen: Absolutely. Here's a favorite recipe of mine for easy-to-prepare Pineapple Salsa. Ingredients:

- 1/2 medium fresh pineapple, peeled and cut into 1/2 inch slices
- 1 small red onion, diced
- 2 jalapeno peppers, seeded and diced
- 2 tablespoons minced fresh cilantro
- 2 tablespoons lime juice

Steve: Combine all the ingredients in a bowl. Refrigerate for 30–60 minutes or until chilled.

Karen: Okay, now I'm really getting hungry.

Steve: Bottom line, guys. If you pig out and are over-stuffed, eat some pineapple. And if you're not stuffed, eat some pineapple anyway. It's great tasting and has some amazing health benefits, including reducing inflammation and aiding in digestion.

Karen: This was a challenging topic.

Steve: I eat challenge for breakfast.

Karen: Yeah, after I make it.

Raspberry – Fruit with a Lisp

Steve: On many a trip to the Pacific Northwest, I've come across wild raspberries growing in the forest, along the side of the road, and even in people's front yards.

Karen: Not so common down here in Southern California.

Steve: No, it isn't. And that's too bad because wild raspberries are so fresh and flavorful.

Karen: We have, however, found some delicious raspberries at the farmer's market, and even on occasion at the grocery store.

Steve: Yes, we have.

Karen: Let's talk about the health benefits of the raspberry. Not only are they delicious, they are remarkably high in fiber. A full cup has over 8 grams of fiber, that's more than you'll get from most boxed cereals!

Steve: Even if you eat the cereal and the box.

Karen: Raspberries contain powerful antioxidants. As a reminder, we need all the antioxidants we can get in order to fight free radicals, which can break down our body tissue. An example of this is the breakdown of collagen and elastin fibers that leads to loss of skin elasticity and wrinkles.

Steve: Ah, wrinkles. Nature's tiny skin moguls.

Karen: As I was saying, raspberries are extremely rich in nutrients that give us protection against free radical damage. These nutrients include vitamin C, manganese, and quercetin. Research published in the *Journal of Agriculture and Food Chemistry* suggests that raspberries may even prevent Cancer. In studies, researchers found that raspberries may inhibit Cancer cells from spreading.

Steve: Yep.

Karen: You're still thinking about the rusty car analogy, aren't you?

Steve: You know me too well.

Karen: Try to keep up. As an added bonus, a full cup of raspberries is only 60 calories, about a quarter of the calories you would find in some nutrition bars. Think about that next time you reach for a snack.

Steve: I hate rust.

Karen: Train's down the track and you're still on the platform.

Steve: Okay, back and focused.

Karen: When you buy raspberries, it's important that they're fresh and ripe.

Steve: Like grapefruits and pineapples, they will not ripen after they have been picked.

Karen: When you buy raspberries, make sure they have deep color and are plump. No plump jokes.

Steve: Wouldn't think of it.

Karen: You also want to avoid raspberries that are soft and mushy. No soft and mushy jokes.

Steve: Plump, soft and mushy, why would I joke about that?

Karen: Because I know you.

Steve: I'm changing my ways.

Karen: Raspberries are highly perishable so you want to eat them within 3 days of purchase.

Steve: Okay, I have a song for new parents. It's called "Plump, Soft and Mushy — Look What Came Out of My Son's Tushy."

Karen: I knew it!

Steve: Okay, now we can move on.

Karen: When considering organic versus non-organic raspberries, it's important to note that pesticides tend to linger on this berry. Buy organic raspberries whenever possible.

Steve: If you want to work raspberries into your diet, think of them as snacks. Also, toss fresh or frozen berries into yogurt, oatmeal, or cereals, especially if you're eating a cereal with low fiber because we know what fiber does!

Karen: Yes, we do. It's becoming a "regular" topic.

Steve: Hey, that was good!

Karen: Here's something you may want to try when you have a sweet tooth. Take some Greek yogurt, add a little honey, or stevia, top with raspberries, and sprinkle with pine nuts.

Steve: Another one of my favorites.

Karen: Make a salad using raspberries, watermelon, and fresh mint. This makes an excellent side dish or dessert. And raspberries go really well on spinach salads.

Steve: Okay, you're up to bat for the bottom line time.

Karen: Bottom line, gentlemen. Raspberries pack a powerful punch when it comes to fighting free radical damage and delivering fiber. They're also loaded with nutrients such as vitamin C, manganese, and quercetin. Eat some. Enjoy some. And eat some more.

Steve: C'mon. Admit it. You liked the song title.

Karen: Actually, it was pretty funny.

Steve: Maybe I should write the lyrics.

Karen: Not that funny.

For a boatload of healthy product suggestions, visit:
IMarriedaNutritionist.com
Click on "Karen's Selections."

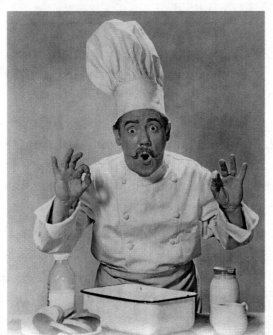

THE COOKING STUFF

CHAPTER 5

"Cooking is like love. It should be entered into with abandon or not at all."
~ Harriet Van Horne

"I think Harriet makes a good point. But where was she when I was single?"
~ Steve Roth

Remembering Where You Put the Coconut Oil

Steve: Someone once said that the only good thing about Alzheimer's is that you never have to watch reruns on TV. Although that may be true, Alzheimer's is certainly nothing to take lightly. The disease afflicts over 5.4 million people in the US, one-in-eight older Americans, and is our sixth leading cause of death.

Karen: Mary T. Newport, MD, medical director of the neo-natal intensive care unit at Spring Hill Regional Hospital in Florida, knows a lot about Alzheimer's Disease.

Steve: Does she ever.

Karen: Her husband came down with Alzheimer's, and when the usual suspects of pharmaceutical drugs proved little help for her husband's condition, she took matters into her own hands and did some serious research.

Steve: I love proactive people. They're just so ... proactive like.

Karen: Dr. Newport discovered that with Alzheimer's Disease, certain brain cells may have difficulty using glucose which is made from the carbs we eat and which is our brain's main source of energy.

Steve: Without fuel, our brain's neurons begin to die.

Karen: Digging further, Dr. Newport learned that there's an alternative energy source for brain cells known as ketones, which the body produces when you consume medium-chain triglyceride oils.

Steve: Otherwise known as MCTs.

Karen: Okay, now here's where it gets really interesting.

Steve: Way to build up the suspense.

Karen: Dr. Newport uncovered that the ingredient that was showing so much promise in drug trials was none other than MCT oil, which is derived from coconut oil.

Steve: Coconut oil?

Karen: That's right. According to the latest research, coconut oil not only protects against Alzheimer's but may actually reverse it!

Steve: Check you out. I didn't know that!

Karen: Yes, you did.

Steve: Okay, I did know that because I'm married to a nutritionist. However, I wanted to sound surprised to further build the excitement.

Karen: No need to build further excitement. This is exciting news. And the good news doesn't stop there. Coconut oil may also benefit people with Parkinson's Disease, Huntington's Disease, Multiple Sclerosis, ALS/Lou Gehrig's Disease, Drug-Resistant Epilepsy, Brittle Type 1 Diabetes, and Type 2 (insulin resistant) Diabetes.

Steve: Wait a minute. If that's true, why haven't more people heard about it?

Karen: The answer is simple. Coconut oil can't be patented and there's no incentive for pharmaceutical companies to promote it.

Steve: You gotta be kidding.

Karen: I wish I were.

Steve: I guess it's the same reason pharmaceutical companies aren't interested in developing a Malaria drug.

Karen: Exactly. There's no paying market for it. But that's where non-profits like the Gates Foundation come in.

Steve: Yes. We saw the story on *60 Minutes*. The Gates Foundation is pouring money into its own research for a Malaria drug for the simple reason of helping save lives, not profit.

Karen: Unfortunately, that's often how the system works. Okay, now back to Dr. Newport's husband.

Steve: The unfortunate guy with Alzheimer's.

Karen: Yes. He began taking coconut oil twice a day and soon showed signs of steady improvement. Over the next year, the Dementia continued to reverse itself and an MRI showed that the brain atrophy had been completely halted. Where synthetic Alzheimer's drugs had failed, a natural substance, coconut oil, seemed to show promise.

Steve: This is big stuff.

Karen: Yes, it is.

Steve: Now I'm sure a lot of our readers will want to learn more about this.

Karen: And they can if they visit Dr. Newport's website at: Coconutketones.com

Steve: Coconut oil can be found in both health food stores and many mainstream grocery stores.

Karen: I recommend getting organic, extra-virgin, cold-pressed coconut oil that's not refined, deodorized, or bleached.

Steve: Bleached?

Karen: Unfortunately, some are. At our house, we cook many of our foods in coconut oil. It's not only incredibly healthy for you but it makes your food taste great and house smell fantastic!

Steve: And don't forget to mention that *coconut oil* is very heat-stable, which makes it perfect for cooking at high temperatures like frying.

Karen: Bottom line, gentlemen …

Steve: Wait, my turn. You did the last one.

Karen: But it's a new chapter.

Steve: Basketball games don't start over in the second half. Score continues.

Karen: That was a weak analogy.

Steve: But one our guy readers can relate to.

Karen: I think you need to give the guys a little more credit.

Steve: Bottom line, guys. Put aside your vegetable oil and give coconut oil a try. It'll lube your food like no

other, smell great, allow you to kick up the burners, and it supports optimum health.

Karen: Bravo. An amazing bottom line. Perhaps the best one of this chapter.

Steve: This is the first one.

Karen: I rest my case.

Sea Salt versus Table Salt Knockdown

Steve: We humans just love salt. It's cheap and it enhances the taste of food.

Karen: For that reason, everything from restaurant food to packaged foods and beverages are loaded with salt.

Steve: That's why Karen and I choose to limit our eating out and eat fresh food at home whenever possible. Okay, here's the stats.

Karen: Why are you looking at me?

Steve: You're the stats person. Remember, I tee it up.

Karen: How about I write down the first statistic about salt and you read it.

Steve: That'll work.

Karen: Here.

Steve: I can't read it.

Karen: Why?

Steve: Your handwriting is terrible. Maybe you should try printing.

Karen: And maybe you should try remembering the stats, such as a healthy adult should consume no more than 1,500 to 2,300 milligrams of sodium per day.

Steve: I knew that.

Karen: Selective memory, right?

Steve: A healthy adult should consume no more than 1,500 to 2,300 milligrams of sodium per day. Exceed that and you're asking for health problems, everything from high blood pressure to heartburn.

Karen: You see? You were good.

Steve: Thank you.

Karen: Good at repeating what I say.

Steve: Okay, well how about this? When you buy salt, you have several options including the traditional table salt … and sea salt.

Karen: Both are made up of sodium and chloride. The big difference between the two is texture, taste, amount of processing, and where it comes from.

Steve: Table salt from land. Sea salt from?

Karen: Outer space.

Steve: You were supposed to say the ocean.

Karen: Precisely.

Steve: Let's look at table salt first. It's what most people have on their tables, thus the name, "table salt." Although, I suppose if you kept your table salt on the counter all the time, it could be called "counter salt."

Karen: But since there are more tables than counters …

Steve: My point exactly. I was getting there.

Karen: Table salt, which comes from underground salt deposits, is much more processed than sea salt, and it has additives such as calcium silicate which keeps it from clumping together in humidity. Table salt is chemically treated and can be bitter tasting.

Steve: Table salt also has added iodine, something that started in the 1920s to help fight a medical condition called Goiter. I hate the name of that condition. Sounds so …

Karen: Goiterish?

Steve: I'm not sure, but I do know I never want it. Your thyroid swells up and makes your neck look like you swallowed a softball. In addition to looking bad and feeling bad, Goiter stretches the hell out of your turtlenecks.

Karen: You certainly have a way with words.

Steve: Thank you.

Karen: Sea salt, on the other hand, is generally considered the healthier salt. It's made by evaporating sea water, which leaves behind natural minerals that give sea salt color and flavor. Those minerals, which are good for your system, include iron, sulphur, and magnesium.

Steve: Let me guess. These minerals are removed during the table-salt-making process?

Karen: You guessed right. If used in moderation, again under the 2,300 milligrams per day, sea salt can be beneficial to your circulatory system by regulating irregular heartbeats and high blood pressure. And get this. Sea salt has also been found to reduce the incidence of Heart Disease and heart attacks.

Steve: Salt helping with Heart Disease?

Karen: If used in moderation.

Steve: Let's turn the focus up the nose.

Karen: Excuse me?

Steve: Sea salt is great for clearing sinus cavities since it's a natural antihistamine.

Karen: That was a strange transition.

Steve: Call me Dr. Strange, Love.

Karen: If you're an athlete, it's important to know that sea salt helps maintain a proper balance of electrolytes in the body, which can strengthen your immune system and increase energy levels.

Steve: And guys, while you're admiring your muscular physique in the mirror, know that sea salt helps improve muscle tone and strength, and helps prevent muscle cramps.

Karen: After a day of exercise, sea salt can help regulate your sleep. In fact, drinking a pinch of sea salt with warm water before turning in can help promote deep sleep.

Steve: You are getting sleepy … sleepy. Look at my watch.

Karen: You look at your watch. I have a bottom line to do. Bottom line, gentlemen. Try switching from regular table salt to sea salt. It's much healthier for you, tastes better, and promotes good health.

Steve: Plus it sounds better in a group when you say, "Pass the sea salt." Very Jacques Cousteau!

Cayenne – Red, Hot and Sprinkly

Steve: Ah, the cayenne. Zero to sixty in 4.6 seconds.

Karen: Is that what cayenne does to you? Zoom. Zoom. Zoom.

Steve: No, that's Mazda. A whole different price range.

Karen: Then what does this have to do with cayenne pepper?

Steve: Pepper? I was talking about the Porsche Cayenne. That sporty SUV that makes suburban moms shiver and suburban dads reclaim their manhood.

Karen: How about we talk seasonings and leave the car review to *Car and Driver?*

Steve: But I'm interested in test-driving a Cayenne.

Karen: And I would like to talk about cayenne pepper. I win because that's what this book is about … nutrition and not skid marks.

Steve: And if you eat healthy, you may not have to deal with skid marks. So there.

Karen: Let's not go there. Did you know that the seasonings you use on your food can have health benefits? Cayenne and other red chili peppers have been shown to reduce cholesterol and triglyceride levels. Cayenne also has a high concentration of a substance called capsaicin. This substance is what gives it the heat. And it's been widely studied for its cardiovascular benefits.

Steve: And if you're a lover of spicy peppers, you know how they can open up congested nasal passages.

Karen: The capsaicin in peppers is similar to a compound found in many over-the-counter decongestants.

Steve: But, as we know, food is a more natural way to handle nasal congestion than drugs, and in this case, capsaicin works much faster. Feel the rush! Oh, yeah.

Karen: Sipping a tea made with hot cayenne pepper will very quickly stimulate the mucus membranes lining the nasal passages and cause drainage, helping relieve congestion and stuffiness.

Steve: Next time you get a cold, give it a try. I have and it works. This also makes a great liquid to gargle with if you have a sore throat. The pepper "burns away" the pain, numbing it out and killing the virus! Hi-Yah!

Karen: Did you just karate kick a virus?

Steve: I did, indeed.

Karen: One additional benefit you can receive from eating hot peppers such as cayenne is that they can boost your metabolism. That heat that you feel after eating something hot actually takes calories to produce, so this is a great seasoning to use if you're trying to lose weight.

Steve: Cayenne pepper adds zest and heat to many dishes. You can control the heat by lightly dusting your food. Try sprinkling cayenne on any stir-fry dishes, stews, and chilies.

Karen: Keep a shaker of cayenne on the table next to the salt and pepper so it's handy.

Steve: That works. Spice up a can of boring beans by adding chopped onions and tomatoes and sprinkle with cayenne. What a perfect side dish for your next Mexican meal.

Karen: Better yet, sprinkle cayenne on baked potatoes, or slices of jicama or cucumbers.

Steve: How about cayenne on scrambled eggs or even deviled eggs?

Karen: You can even mix it into dips, such as guacamole or salsa.

Steve: We have to stop here.

Karen: Why?

Steve: I'm getting incredibly hungry. **Bottom line, guys.**
Cayenne gets the blood flowing, helps relieve congestion and stuffiness, kicks up your metabolism, and is
a tasty spice for a whole variety of foods. Experiment.
You might just find all kinds of foods to improve with a
little kick.

Mr. Stinky – Garlic

Steve: Okay, guys. Here's a very bold statement. Garlic is one of the healthiest foods you can eat.

Karen: Check you out. Going all bold on us.

Steve: What?

Karen: That was a very bold statement and you said it with such conviction.

Steve: Well, you know how much I like garlic.

Karen: Do I ever. Phew.

Steve: C'mon, you're a big garlic fan, too.

Karen: Okay, I confess. I am. And that's why we try to always eat garlic together.

Steve: A good practice for any couple.

Karen: Regular consumption of garlic has been shown to lower blood pressure, decrease triglycerides and LDL cholesterol, all while elevating HDL cholesterol.

Steve: Yet another food we've introduced that lowers triglycerides.

Karen: I'm hoping everyone is putting this all together that diet, in many cases, can do as much or more than pharmaceuticals in improving cholesterol.

Steve: You mean controlling cholesterol.

Karen: We don't just want to control cholesterol, we want to improve it!

Steve: Which makes this chapter perfect for guys. We improve stuff. Give us the facts, we look at the big picture. If it makes sense, we task it out and make it better.

Karen: I'm glad to hear that.

Steve: And I'm counting on the guys to back me up on this one or I'll have to eat crow.

Karen: That was certainly said with confidence.

Steve: I eat confidence for breakfast ... along with a hard-boiled egg.

Karen: Garlic also contains sulphur compounds that can reduce inflammation which may be contributing to Arthritis or even Asthma.

Steve: Cholesterol, Arthritis, and Asthma. Tell me more, oh bastion of nutritional knowledge.

Karen: These same sulphur compounds that you find in garlic also act as an antibacterial and antiviral agent. It's even believed that regular consumption of garlic can ward off colds.

Steve: Makes sense. It's known to ward off vampires and evil spirits.

Karen: Let's stick to reality, okay?

Steve: Don't want to mess with vampires. That's involuntary blood donation.

Karen: Here's something you might find interesting, Mister Vampire Authority. There was a study done using allicin, a phytonutrient found in garlic, where animals were divided into three groups and all were given the same diet. The two groups receiving the allicin with their food either maintained their body weight or actually lost a little weight, while the group not given allicin gained weight.

Steve: So the allicin in garlic may help with weight loss?

Karen: According to the study, yes. Now, when buying garlic, you want to give the bulb a gentle squeeze to test for firmness.

Steve: I think the guys can relate to that.

Karen: And you don't want to feel softness.

Steve: Absolutely not. Like pushing a rope up hill.

Karen: And you don't want dampness in the bulb.

Steve: Quick. Grab the tissue.

Karen: And when it comes to storing garlic, it's best to keep it in a cool, dark, dry place for up to a month.

Steve: And you don't want to store garlic in the refrigerator. Why? Tee up.

Karen: Because it will cause the garlic to sprout and taste bitter. However, if it does sprout, that doesn't mean you have to throw it out.

Steve: Absolutely not. You can still eat garlic that's sprouted; it will just have a slight bitter taste.

Karen: Now, once you pull off a garlic clove, remember that it speeds up the garlic's shelf life. So try to use the rest of the garlic within a couple of weeks.

Steve: I didn't know that. Although it does make sense.

Karen: You can add fresh pressed garlic to dips like hummus or guacamole. Stir it into mashed potatoes. I use minced garlic in all my stir-fry dishes.

Steve: Does she ever.

Karen: And when I cook something in the Crock-Pot, I always toss in a few whole garlic cloves.

Steve: Sometimes I do that from across the room, although I try not to dunk. That can make a mess.

Karen: Bottom line, gentlemen. Garlic makes everything taste better, and it's amazingly good for you, from helping lower cholesterol, to reducing inflammation, to helping prevent weight gain.

Steve: Okay, guys. You heard the lowdown on garlic. You know what to do.

Karen: What's that?

Steve: Get stinky!

Dressing and Undressing Salad Dressing

Karen: We're now going to talk about salad dressing.

Steve: And undressing …

Karen: … the salad dressing.

Steve: Have you noticed that people seem to be eating a lot of salads these days?

Karen: Yes, I have noticed that.

Steve: I have a theory about it.

Karen: Well, don't leaf us hanging. Lettuce begin.

Steve: Hey, that was pretty good. A bit corny, but well done.

Karen: Thank you. I've been watching how you add humor to the book.

Steve: And you're copying it?

Karen: Actually, I'm trying to do better. He just shot me a look. Just kidding! Okay, Humor Man, share your theory with us.

Steve: I think people are eating more salads for three reasons.

Karen: Can a theory have three reasons?

Steve: According to Albert Einstein, yes. Just don't ask me to quote him. Okay, here's what I think. First, more and more restaurants are offering salads, from basic salads at fast food joints, to more exotic entrée salads at sit-down restaurants. It's becoming fashionable to eat salad.

Karen: I'll agree with that.

Steve: Second, people are becoming more health-conscious and making healthier choices when eating out.

Karen: Makes sense.

Steve: Third, there's the growing popularity of stores such as Whole Foods, Sprouts, Trader Joe's, Henry's and Lassen's, whose culture is to promote healthy food options, including organic fruits and vegetables.

Karen: I would add that mainstream grocers, such as Albertsons and Jewel-Osco, are also emphasizing their fresh produce in their advertising.

Steve: Yes, they are.

Karen: Can I add to your theory?

Steve: Absolutely, my theory buddy.

Karen: Farmer's markets are becoming very popular across the country, and people are being exposed to all sorts of delicious local produce. In addition, in this economy, people are discovering how cost-effective and fun it can be to grow your own vegetables and fruit, like we're doing in our backyard.

Steve: Having your own vegetable garden is a great way to get kids interested in vegetables and fruit. Somehow it always tastes better when you grow it yourself.

Karen: I totally agree. Now when it comes to preparing your salad, a lot of people don't realize that they may be sabotaging their health with what they put on their salad. Many of the salad dressings you buy in the store contain MSG and hydrogenated oils.

Steve: Monosodium glutamate (MSG) is a flavor enhancer that the Food and Drug Administration (FDA) has classified a food ingredient that's "generally recognized as safe." However, some people experience adverse reactions to foods containing MSG, including headaches, sweating, flushing, numbness, chest pain, nausea, and weakness.

Karen: Gee, sounds like something I want on my salad.

Steve: Luckily the FDA requires all foods containing MSG to list it on the label.

Karen: Another thing about salad dressings, and many packaged foods for that matter, is that when a product is labeled "fat free" it usually contains a significant amount of sugar and way too much sodium.

Steve: There's that darn hidden sugar again.

Karen: Exactly. When the fat is removed, a lot of the flavor goes away and food manufacturers try to replace that flavor with sugar and salt.

Steve: Very sneaky.

Karen: Keeping in mind that the serving size for most salad dressings is 2 tablespoons, I'm going to share some numbers with you.

Steve: Two tablespoons. Lock and load. Go.

Karen: A typical ranch dressing will cost you 100 calories, 11 grams of fat, and 300 milligrams of sodium.

Steve: Considering the recommended daily amount of sodium for an adult is 1,500 to 2,300 milligrams, that's a lot.

Karen: Yes, it is. Typical blue cheese dressing will be double that at 200 calories, 20 grams of fat, and the same amount of sodium … *if* you use only 2 tablespoons.

Steve: Big IF. Even I have a hard time limiting the amount of salad dressing I use. I think it's a guy thing. We coat our salads the way we paint a wall. Put it on thick so you only need one coat.

Karen: Women tend to do the same thing, we're just more conscious of our calorie intake.

Steve: Okay, so say I'm using "fat free" or "light" dressing …

Karen: Light dressing may be low in calories, but it often contains high fructose corn syrup and a lot of sodium.

Steve: Jeez. Everywhere you turn, there's a landmine.

Karen: And don't be fooled by dressings you spray on your salad. They may contain multiple preservatives that can be dangerous to your health. I even saw a honey mustard flavor spray-on dressing that contained Yellow Dye #5 and artificial flavors along with preservatives. You're totally sabotaging your salad with that!

Steve: Fortunately, when Karen points out problems, she also provides solutions.

Karen: Your best option is to simply use olive oil and your favorite vinegar, or make your own concoction. One of our favorites is: ½ cup coconut vinegar, ½ cup coconut aminos, olive oil to taste (optional).

Steve: If that's too much work for you guys, go to our website at IMarriedaNutritionist.com and click on the "Karen's Selections" tab for a list of healthy salad dressings we use when we don't make our own. Many of the products we recommend have small marketing budgets and fight for shelf space at grocers. But if it's a great product, we feel it's our responsibility to let you know about it. If your store doesn't carry it, oftentimes you can order it on the company's website or ask your grocer to stock it!

Karen: Many of these healthy salad dressings can also be used as marinades.

Steve: Bottom line, guys. Don't turn healthy salads into high-calorie and high-fat meals. Be aware of what's in the dressing you're putting on your salad. You wouldn't put a snow suit on a bathing suit model, would you?

Karen: What if it was cold outside and she was shivering?

Steve: You make a good point … and I'm guessing she would, too.

Karen: Unfortunately you wouldn't! High-five!

This Barbecue Rub
Leads to a Happy Ending

Steve: Okay, here's the rub …

Karen: That was so expected.

Steve: Well, they can't all be gems.

Karen: Apparently not.

Steve: Why are you staring at me?

Karen: I've never noticed this before but from the side, you sort of look like Tim Allen.

Steve: Yes, I've heard that before.

Karen: I mean, not exactly, but there is some resemblance.

Steve: Yes, because if I looked exactly like him, I would have to carry around a pen and sign autographs.

Karen: You would do that?

Steve: Sure. You can't disappoint the fans.

Karen: So, would you sign your name or his?

Steve: Why are you so interested in this?

Karen: I think it reveals a lot about you.

Steve: I would sign my name, but scribble it so it could be his name if somebody didn't know what his name looked like.

Karen: I see. All because you didn't want to disappoint anyone?

Steve: Correct. Life's full of disappointments. Who am I to add one more to the list?

Karen: Interesting.

Steve: And if I don't get back to this barbecue rub, our readers are going to be disappointed.

Karen: Nice segue.

Steve: Thank you. I wrote it myself. Now, when it comes to steaks, let them sit at room temperature for 25–30 minutes before grilling. This shortens the cooking time; the interior of each steak reaches its desired doneness faster, so there's less chance of overcooking the exterior.

Karen: Tell us more about the recipe, Man Who Looks Like Tim Allen from the side.

Steve: This recipe makes enough rub for four steaks. If you want, double the recipe and store half for your next barbecue.

Karen: Brilliant! Sheer brilliance!

Steve: Hold your applause until the end. Okay, here's the rub:

- 2 teaspoons sea salt
- ½ tablespoon pepper
- ½ teaspoon garlic powder
- ½ teaspoon oregano
- ½ teaspoon thyme
- ½ teaspoon paprika
- ¼ teaspoon cayenne pepper

Karen: All healthy ingredients.

Steve: Mix all the ingredients in small bowl. Lightly coat the steaks with olive oil, correct?

Karen: You guessed right.

Steve: Next, you want to massage the rub into both sides of your organic, grass-fed steak as if Miss January asked you to rub sunblock on her back poolside at the Playboy Mansion.

Karen: Oh, now there's a visual.

Steve: Just building the added-value fantasy for our guy readers.

Karen: You're a very responsible author.

Steve: I try to be. So, there you have it, a healthy rub for a healthy steak, for a healthy chef, and his three half-naked cheerleaders playing croquet at his Beverly Hills mansion.

Karen: You wish.

Steve: Upon a star! But the reality is, I don't need three half-naked cheerleaders because I married a nutritionist.

Karen: You're stretching it, buddy.

Steve: Well, I was a minute ago. **Bottom line, guys. There's nothing wrong with making your own barbecue rub. It's probably much healthier than what you can buy in the store. Plus you get points for making it yourself!**

Safe Grilling Is Like Safe Sex

Steve: Any good riddle that's properly set up leaves the listener, or in this case, the reader, waiting for the punch line.

Karen: So you're going to tell us a riddle?

Steve: Yes.

Karen: Why the big setup?

Steve: I like to ease into things.

Karen: Okay, so what's the riddle?

Steve: You seem to be in a hurry.

Karen: No hurry, I'm just trying to keep things moving along.

Steve: Fine. How is safe grilling like safe sex?

Karen: I don't know. Your steak doesn't get pregnant?

Steve: The better you plan ahead, the better the meat is for you.

Karen: That's what all the buildup was about?

Steve: Yes.

Karen: Maybe you better subscribe to *Playboy*.

Steve: Ding! Ding! Ding! You see, guys, *that* is how you outsmart your wife to get her to suggest that you subscribe to *Playboy*.

Karen: Oh brother.

Steve: Clever is as clever does.

Karen: Goofy is as goofy does. While you pat yourself on the back, how about I take over? Research shows that cooking food at high heat, especially on a grill, can create carcinogenic compounds to form on your food.

Steve: Are we talking HCAs?

Karen: Yes, heterocyclic amines, otherwise known as HCAs, are created when meat is charbroiled or overcooked.

Steve: And lab animals who ate HCAs at their barbecues have been known to develop Cancer.

Karen: Polycyclic aromatic hydrocarbons (PAHs) are another carcinogen related to grilling. They're created when fat drips from the meat, hits the charcoal or burner, and smokes up on the food.

Steve: Okay, guys, I know what you're thinking. No way am I giving up my barbecuing. And rightfully so. What we're recommending is *grilling smarter.*

Karen: Here are some simple changes to your old barbecuing habits that will be much better for your health.

Steve: According to Kansas State University scientists, using marinades can reduce HCA buildup on your food by an average of 71%.

Karen: Another thing you can do to avoid carcinogens is to slow cook your meat over lower heat. Of course, this is easier if you have a gas grill.

Steve: Flip your meat frequently. And when you're done with that, flip the meat on the grill.

Karen: I don't know how to respond to that.

Steve: In life, some things don't need a response. Here's something else you can do. Trimming the extra fat on the meat will help reduce flare-ups.

Karen: Yeah, it's best to remove that char-thing from your repertoire.

Steve: Oh, and if you've never grilled veggies and fruit, such as sliced eggplant, scallions, squash, and pineapple, give it a try. They're not as susceptible to HCAs and PHAs.

Karen: Bottom line, gentlemen. Grilling can be safe if you follow a few simple rules. Use marinade, cook over a low heat and avoid flair-ups.

Steve: Rules? Our guy readers don't follow rules. They eat them for breakfast!

Karen: I probably shouldn't have mentioned that Tim Allen thing.

Steve: Want an autograph?

Karen: Absolutely.

Steve: Really?

Karen: Here. Sign this blank check.

Shish Kabobs – Stick'em and Lick'em

Steve: The term *"shish kebab"* comes from Turkish words which literally mean "skewer" and "roast meat." It's a signature Turkish meal. Kebabs, or kabobs, were used by nomadic tribes as a convenient way to marinate unusual meats on-the-go to get rid of their gamey flavor. What kind of meats … I don't want to know.

Karen: It is written that Christopher Columbus really got into Portuguese *espetadas*, a beef shish kabob marinated in wine.

Steve: Can't say for sure that the wine was the reason Chris had trouble navigating the high seas and finding the New World, but it's good made-up trivia for your next poker game.

Karen: To begin making shish kabobs, start with either metal or wooden skewers. Metal skewers can be re-used, while wooden skewers can be tossed after use.

Steve: Remember to soak wooden skewers in water before using them, otherwise they'll flame up. Another note about wooden skewers, it's not proper etiquette to use a wooden skewer as a toothpick at the dinner table. It not only makes you look like a hillbilly, but it could lead to oral splinters which are hard to explain at the dentist. Just ask Martha Washington.

Karen: Any kind of meat or seafood you might typically barbecue can be used in shish kabobs … beef, pork, chicken, shrimp, scallops, or fish. Needless to say, we prefer organic meats and wild seafood whenever possible.

Steve: Common vegetables used on the skewer include onions, mushrooms, bell peppers, eggplant, tomatoes, zucchini, and other kinds of squash. If you're adventurous, try adding fruit to your kabobs, such as pineapple and melons.

Karen: You can mix vegetables with meat on the same skewer, or keep the veggies and meat separate. Sometimes separate works better for grilling, if either the meat or vegetables take longer to cook.

Steve: Figure 5 to 7 minutes on each side, and long tongs work best for flipping those babies over.

Karen: If you're planning a backyard barbecue, definitely consider shish kabobs. Your dinner guests will be impressed and they're so easy to prepare.

Steve: And best of all, they're healthy as long as you don't stab yourself with a skewer.

Karen: Like that's going to happen.

Steve: Tailgate party?

Karen: Okay, I see your point.

Steve: Bottom line, guys. Shish kabobs are a healthy meal that's fun and convenient to cook. Plus shish kabobs have the ability to impresses the hell out of friends and neighbors.

Karen: Which I'm guessing most guys like to do.

Steve: Goes back to caveman days, I'm sure. "Hey, Rocky. Get a load of this Cryolophosaurus and zucchini combo on a stick!"

Karen: Cryolophosaurus?

Steve: You don't know about the Cryolophosaurus? It was a dinosaur once known as "Elvisaurus" due to the crest on its head which looked like Elvis' pompadour.

Karen: You're making that up.

Steve: Google it. I did. He ain't nothin' like a hound dog, is he Riley? You're the hound dog, Buddy.

Crock-Pot Recipe – That's Not a Bunch of Crock

Steve: I was watching Karen whip up one of our favorite dinners the other day, and I said, "We just have to share this with the guys."

Karen: Absolutely. This is just too simple and too much of a time-saver not to get the word out.

Steve: If you don't know much about Crock-Pots, well, they can be your best friend. They listen to you when you're down, or drunk … like Tom Hanks and that volleyball. You can lean on it, just make sure it's not too hot. And it makes amazing meals that make your house smell good for 2 days, especially if you have gas.

Karen: Had to throw that in, didn't you?

Steve: There was a reason for it. If you eat out at restaurants a lot, there's a decent chance you'll get gas. Restaurant food can be tough on your system and your system sometimes fights back with a booty bomb … a bratwurst boogie … or a tush tickler.

Karen: You can justify anything, can't you?

Steve: Pretty much.

Karen: Although there are many great Crock-Pot recipes, this is one of my favorites. Healthy. Delicious. Easy to prepare. Crock-Pot Chicken. Here are the ingredients:

- 1 whole organic, free-range chicken
- 2 medium sweet potatoes
- 2 onions
- 4 carrots
- Mushrooms and a variety of greens, such as collard, mustard or kale (optional)

- ▶ Seasoning mixture:
  - 1 tablespoon olive oil
  - 1 teaspoon paprika
  - I teaspoon of each: thyme, basil, salt, garlic powder, and pepper

Steve: First, you cut up the carrots, potatoes, and onions into big chunks, which you layer across the bottom of the Crock-Pot. Consider it a bed for your bird.

Karen: Then take your chicken, rinse it off in the sink, and wipe it dry with paper towels.

Steve: At this point, you can have some optional fun with your chicken, just don't drop it on the floor. Grab your chicken … but don't choke your chicken. That's never acceptable in the kitchen. Throw the chicken in the air to do a 2½ flip, then make it moon walk across the countertop while you sing a song from the *Thriller* album. Stick a potato in its head hole and do the old Mister Potato Head routine with some tooth-picks and two olives. When you're done being a guy, make sure you thoroughly wash every surface with soap and water that came in contact with the raw chicken … including you!

Karen: I think I'm going to take my name off this book.

Steve: Really? Okay, maybe I went a little far with the Mister Potato Head bit.

Karen: Place your chicken in the Crock-Pot on top of the carrots, potatoes, and onions.

Steve: Breast side up, gentlemen. Uh-oh. She just gave me the warning look.

Karen: Rub the seasoning mix on the chicken and cover the Crock-Pot. Let it cook on low for 8-9 hours. If you're around one-hour before the chicken is done, place a few handfuls of the greens around the chicken. If you like mushrooms, add those as well at that time. Never put these in at the beginning or they'll turn into mush! They only need about an hour to cook down.

Steve: When all is said and done, you'll most likely have some great leftovers!

Karen: Bottom line, gentlemen. For a busy person, Crock-Pots are terrific. Assemble everything the night before, put the Crock-Pot in the refrigerator, and simply plug it in before you go to work, hit the ski slopes, or head out on the golf course. When you get home, you'll have an instant dinner waiting.

Steve: Very nice wrap-up.

Karen: Had to do something to counterbalance your playing with the chicken routine.

Steve: What? The chicken doesn't care. It's his 5 minutes of fame.

Karen: Or embarrassment.

Steve: What do you mean?

Karen: What if another chicken walked by and saw what you were doing? It would be all over the hen house.

Steve: What other chicken? The one in the freezer? And we don't have a hen house.

Karen: Okay, then say Riley walked in the kitchen and saw what you were doing. He might think he was next.

Steve: Now you're just being silly. Riley knows only one trick and that's how to sit. There's no way he could ever moon walk.

Karen: You don't know that. He might be holding back on us.

Steve: I think I'm ready to close this out.

Karen: Or, maybe an Elvisaurus might walk by and see what you were doing with the chicken. What then?

Steve: I get your point. No playing with the chicken.

Karen: Thank you.

Hit the Road Microwave

Steve: Before Karen and I moved into our new place, we were packing up our old kitchen and she said to me, "We need to get rid of this microwave." Looked perfectly good to me. I mean, it's not like we used it a lot, mainly quick heat-ups and such. Then it hit me. She probably wants a new one to match our new refrigerator.

Karen: I told him we were getting rid of the microwave to protect the food we eat.

Steve: Like a skilled lawyer, she began to present her case.

Karen: Microwaves heat food by creating violent friction in the water molecules which eventually turn into steam and warm the food. As the molecules are literally blown apart, the molecular damage spreads beyond the water and into your food, literally changing your food's chemical structure.

Steve: But it didn't stop there.

Karen: Absolutely. A good lawyer presents a complete case before resting. Recent research shows that microwaves significantly decrease the nutritional value of food, so all your good intentions of buying fresh and healthy food can go out the window with microwaving.

Steve: Of course, I immediately starting thinking about all the money we had blown. We had been buying some really good, clean, fresh food, and then destroying it in the microwave.

Karen: Research shows that microwaves reduce levels of vitamin B12, decreases flavonoids in food by 97%, and significantly alters levels of vitamins and nutrients.

Steve: See what I was up against? She had the goods and she delivered them with a razor-sharp prosecution of the microwave.

Karen: And let's say you have a baby at home and breast milk is being heated in a microwave. By doing so, bacteria-digesting enzymes in the breast milk are being broken down and the antibody levels in the milk are being decreased. Oh, and if plastic baby bottles are heated in the microwave, dangerous toxins may be leached into the breast milk or formula.

Steve: The Nazis are credited with inventing the microwave oven. The experimental contraption was used in mobile food support when they invaded the Soviet Union during World War II. Although the US did some research after the war to see just how safe microwave ovens were, it was the Russians who took the lead and, based on their research on the biological effects of microwaving food, they banned the use of microwaves in 1976. The ban was later lifted during Perestroika.

Karen: The Russian investigators found that carcinogens were formed from the microwaving of nearly all foods tested, from milk and grains to frozen fruits, vegetables, and meats. Structural degradation, which decreased food value, was found to be 60-90% overall for foods tested.

Steve: Hard to believe our country wasn't aware of these findings. Then again, it's hard to put the brakes on a new appliance that would revolutionize the food industry.

Karen: So back to the new house and life without a microwave. Surprisingly, it hasn't been a big change in our routine. Liquids heat within 2-3 minutes in a sauce pan on the stove, and stay hot longer. We now heat leftovers in a convection oven, which takes a bit longer than a microwave, but it works perfectly fine if you plan ahead instead of rushing last minute.

Steve: As for frozen foods, pop them in a convection or regular oven and set the timer. Gives you time to have a glass of wine and chill out.

Karen: Before dinner, not breakfast.

Steve: It's five o'clock somewhere in the world. **Bottom line, guys. Your microwave may be destroying the nutritional value of that expensive food you're buying and making it carcinogenic. That's like bringing your date back to your place for the first time and asking her to put on your mother's house dress.**

Karen: Ewe. That was just plain weird.

Steve: No kidding. I think I just weirded myself out.

Karen: You might need a time out for that one.

Steve: Yeah, time out for a gluten-free beer.

For a boatload of healthy product suggestions, visit:
IMarriedaNutritionist.com
Click on "Karen's Selections."

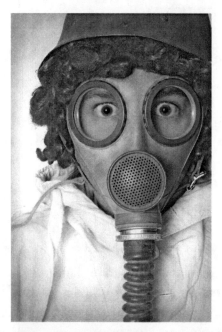

THE TOXIC STUFF

CHAPTER 6

*"Sometimes a toxic person is toxic without knowing it." ~ **Anonymous***

*"Toxic is as toxic does." ~ **Steve Roth***

Sidestepping a Toxic Life

Karen: Most everyone will agree that we live in a very toxic world. Plastics, chemicals, pesticides, and polluted air are just a few of the toxins we interact with in our everyday lives.

Steve: But the good news is that with proper awareness of the toxins in your life you can clean up your act in a very positive way.

Karen: This entire section of the book is all about toxins. But we're going to kick it off slowly with a few simple ideas.

Steve: First up to bat. Your car.

Karen: Tip number one. Let's talk about that intriguing smell of a new car. To many, it signifies something really new and terrific in your life. Well, did you know that your new car smell is simply plastic, leather, and other man-made materials off-gassing?

Steve: Unlike human off-gassing, which can temporarily linger and clear a room if you're really good, the materials in a new car pour toxic vapors 24/7 into your confined driving space for months after you drive it off the lot.

Karen: In California, auto manufacturers are now placing warning stickers on the windows of new cars. My suggestion is when you bring home a new car, air it out as often as possible by leaving the windows down.

Steve: And whether you have a new or old car, air it out before you jump in. A car with its windows rolled up is literally a chamber of floating chemicals. Summer heat accelerates off-gassing and you can often smell it when you slide behind the wheel.

Karen: One last note about your car. When you get it washed, pass on the added fragrance. It's simply more toxins you're pumping into your car, and into your body.

Steve: Tip number two. Your leftovers. If you insist on using a microwave, never heat leftovers in plastic storage containers.

Karen: Take them out of the plastic and put them on a plate that's microwave safe. The heat generated by microwaves causes chemicals in the plastic to leach directly out of the plastic and into your food. An easy solution is to store your leftovers in glass storage containers and put a paper towel over the top when heating.

Steve: Tip number three. Your shower. Plastic shower curtains, especially new ones, off-gas big time, especially with the steam from a hot shower. While you're soapin' and a sudsin' and having a bang up time behind the plastic curtain, you're sucking in some pretty nasty stuff.

Karen: The best solution is to purchase a polyester fabric shower curtain which is water repellant, non-toxic, and doesn't off-gas like vinyl products.

Steve: And finally, tip number four. Take-out coffee. When you buy a cup of take-out coffee, beware of coated paper cups and their plastic lids which often leach chemicals into your coffee.

Karen: It's that heat thing again. Just imagine how hot it gets inside a freshly poured coffee cup. My solution is to buy a stainless-steel coffee mug and take it into Starbucks or any other coffee house and they'll be glad to fill it up ... and the coffee will be cheaper, too!

Steve: Four great tips right off the bat. But, wait, there's more!

Karen: Bottom line, guys. We live in a manufactured world with plenty of toxins, and heat is a big factor in delivering those toxins to you.

Toxic Receipts, Man Boobs and More

Karen: The world produces six billion pounds of the chemical bisphenol A, otherwise known as BPA. It's used in making plastics and a host of other products we use in our everyday lives. It's the plastic part that's been in the news lately.

Steve: You see, when plastic that's made with BPA …

Karen: And that's a lot of the world's plastic …

Steve: Yes, it is. When it's heated, as we discussed in the last section, or if that plastic is stressed, it allows BPA to leach into our food and water.

Karen: We come in contact with BPA in other ways, too. John C. Warner, an organic chemist and co-founder of the Warner Babcock Institute for Green Chemistry, discovered that the amount of BPA on most coated paper receipts can be greater than that found in plastic. It's receipts for credit cards, ATMs, gas pumps, and restaurants. Basically it's all those thin papered receipts we get with the shiny surface on one side.

Steve: Okay, so you're probably thinking, what does BPA do to us? Well, if you're an infant (which you're not, otherwise you wouldn't be reading this), it can be pretty harmful.

Karen: Yes, it can. Exposure to BPA may disrupt the delicate endocrine system in infants, leading to developmental problems. Lots of other ills that have been rising unchecked for a generation, such as Obesity, Diabetes, Autism, and ADD, may also be linked to BPA.

Steve: BPA can mess with your hormones, too. Hormones are one of Karen's areas of expertise.

Karen: BPA can mimic estrogen and mess with testosterone and adrenaline. Tiny amounts of hormones can cause significant biological and behavioral changes.

Steve: For men, that extra estrogen kick can, well, make us girly-like. We're talking mood changes, man boobs, even sterility. When you disrupt your hormones, it can also lead to weight gain and even Cancer.

Karen: Our daily contact with receipts is a big problem. We touch them, put them in our wallets next to our money, and BPA gets onto our hands, on our skin, into our mouths. The chemical spreads everywhere.

Steve: Bottom line, guys. The best thing to do is be conscious of BPA and limit your contact with paper receipts whenever possible. My bank now gives you an option at the ATM to have your receipt emailed to you. Maybe yours does, too. And if you do come in contact with a receipt, remember to wash your hands thoroughly. Otherwise, the next time you're clothes shopping with your wife, you may be eyeing the bra section for reasons other than those sexy mannequins.

Parabens – Different than Pair of Buns

Karen: Hopefully by now you've heard of parabens. They're a group of chemicals used as preservatives in all those personal care products we squirt, lather, scrub, and massage onto our bodies.

Steve: From conditioners on top to sex lube down below, most people are coated with parabens as they are in literally thousands of products used by consumers every day.

Karen: Parabens go by many names such as methylparaben, butylparaben, ethylparaben, benzylparaben, isobutylparaben, and propylparaben. They make it simple for us to remember; just look for any product ingredient ending in "paraben."

Steve: In the 1990s, the scientific community became increasingly aware that some synthetic chemicals were able to interfere with the function of both female and male hormones.

Karen: And within the category of hormone disruptors are xenoestrogens, synthetic chemicals that mimic estrogen. A number of studies have shown that parabens fall into the xenoestrogens' group; xenoestrogens may be linked to high rates of Breast Cancer and reproductive problems in women as well as decreased sperm counts and Prostate and Testicular Cancer in men.

Steve: Product manufacturers and the FDA give a thumbs up to Parabens for consumer use. After all, they give products a long shelf life and they're cheap. However, many people believe more research needs to be done before rubber stamping parabens "safe" for humans and other living things.

Karen: Despite FDA approval, a number of product manufacturers are following consumer demand by removing parabens from some of their products.

Steve: And that's a good thing. Other companies not only ban parabens from their entire product line, but no one within

500 feet of the company headquarters is allowed to say, spell, utter, sing, burp, slur, or hiccup the word "paraben." Actually, I just made that up. No one can hiccup the word "paraben."

Karen: If you have any questions about whether your personal care products contain parabens or any toxic chemicals, go to EWG.org./skindeep.

Steve: As I'm sure you can imagine, with my nutritionist being an expert in hormone imbalance, we're very serious about our home being paraben-free. Again, if you're interested in seeing which products we use and recommend, visit the "Karen's Selections" at IMarriedaNutritionist.com.

Karen: Bottom line, gentlemen. We suggest avoiding parabens whenever possible. It's not just about what goes in your mouth; what goes on your skin and hair is equally as important.

Mercury Fillings – They're a Gas!

Steve: Mercury is one of the most toxic substances on the planet … even more so than the average guy's dirty socks. It can greatly affect the health of your immune, reproductive, neurological, and cardiovascular systems.

Karen: Because mercury has such a profound effect on our nervous system, both in the brain and at cellular level, it has been tied to Parkinson's, Alzheimer's, ALS, and Multiple Sclerosis.

Steve: When you think about mercury toxicity, you immediately think about farmed or contaminated fish. Very few people eat thermometers.

Karen: Steve, I remember you sharing that your mother used to play with mercury from broken thermometers when she was a child. At that time, no one knew the long-term effects of handling mercury. Perhaps that played a role, even a small role, in the chronic illnesses she suffered later in life.

Steve: You may be right. Now here's something interesting. The term "mad as a hatter" from the children's book *Alice in Wonderland* relates to a disease peculiar to the hat making industry in the 1800's. The process of turning fur into felt involved using a mercury solution and when the workers breathed the fumes of this highly toxic metal, it often resulted in symptoms such as trembling, loss of coordination, slurred speech, loosening of teeth, memory loss, depression, irritability and anxiety. It was known as The Mad Hatter Syndrome.

Karen: Which leads us to the mercury that most people come in contact with each and every day without even thinking about it. We're talking about the silver fillings in your mouth. These silver amalgams are at least 50% mercury.

Steve: Since the 1800s, dentists have been putting fillings in people's mouths that are a mix of mercury and other metals.

Karen: According to *HealthKeepers Magazine,* the FDA recently changed its website to say, "High levels of mercury vapor exposure are associated with adverse effects in the brain and the kidneys." Prior to this, the agency's website did not explain to consumers the damage caused by mercury fillings. Hundreds of millions of people have received amalgam fillings, although their popularity has dropped off in recent years. Currently, only about 30% of dental fillings contain mercury – the rest are resin composites made from glass, cement, and porcelain. They're not quite as durable as amalgam and a bit more expensive but they're so much safer for you.

Steve: There's an amazing video on YouTube which demonstrates what we're talking about. Search "Smoking Tooth = Poison Gas." This is the first-ever photography which shows the mercury vapors coming off an old filling. And this is just one filling. Imagine the toxicity you're facing with a mouthful of silver fillings.

Karen: Not all dentists will agree to discuss the dangers of mercury. Like the FDA, their governing body, the American Dental Association, isn't exactly behind admitting to the public that what has been put in your mouth could cause harm.

Steve: After thoroughly researching the issue, Karen and I had all our silver fillings removed. I sleep better at night knowing that the only gas I'm creating is out the other end.

Karen: Not all dentists are equipped to safely remove toxic silver fillings. Protective measures must be in place for both the patient and the dentist. Do your homework if you decide to have your silver fillings removed. Look for a dentist who operates a mercury-free practice, or who advertises herself/

himself as a holistic dentist.

Steve: Bottom line, guys. When getting new fillings, insist on composite materials. As for your old fillings, if you decide to have them removed, seek out a qualified holistic dentist.

Is That a Cell Phone in Your Pocket Or ...

Steve: I recently discovered that every time I put my iPhone in my pants pocket, I'm violating Apple's safety warning.

Karen: Busted!

Steve: I was also doing that when I had my Blackberry.

Karen: Busted again! Two strikes.

Steve: Most people don't know about a related warning that smartphone manufacturers state in their owner's manuals. For your own safety, they say that you should keep your cell phone a certain distance from your body when sending or receiving data in order to "maintain compliance" with radio frequency-radiation standards set by the FCC.

Karen: For Blackberry owners, that safe distance is almost an inch (0.98") while Apple's iPhone 4 manual tells users to keep the phone "at least 5/8 inches away from your body." Motorola? They suggest that an active WI80 should be a full inch from the user's skin, unless it's paired with a company-approved "clip, holder, holster, case, or body harness."

Steve: Now, if you're like most guys who don't read their phone's directions, you're probably keeping your phone in your front pants pocket ... not to replace your rolled-up sock, but for simple convenience. Hey, not everyone can pull off the style of carrying a cell phone clipped to the belt.

Karen: As mentioned in a *Time* magazine article, skeptics of cell phone safety have brushed off the warnings saying that guidelines set in 2001 say cell phone usage is safe. Problem is, all the tests were done with belt clips or holsters. The FCC told testers to assume a distance of 0.59 to 0.98 inches from the body.

Steve: Why should you guys be concerned with this? Because radio-frequency waves can heat cells in your body. So, if you're a guy who puts his cell phone in his right pocket and happen to "dress right," well, you may be cooking sausage without all the trimmings.

Karen: You have an amazing way with words.

Steve: Thank you.

Karen: Think about how many men sometimes put their cell phone in their shirt pocket next to their heart. Or the women who tuck their cell phone in their bra.

Steve: That one I hadn't heard about. "Excuse me, ma'am, but your right breast is ringing."

Karen: Unfortunately it's not long distance, its close distance.

Steve: You got it. Now, the FCC says the link between cell phone exposure and Cancer is inconclusive. Meanwhile, the FDA says it can not rule out the possibility of a health risk from cell phones but if it does exist, it's probably small. However, one recent multi-country study found that people who used their phones on average 30 or more minutes a day for 10 years had a substantially higher risk of developing Brain Cancer.

Karen: That's of course holding a phone to your ear, not using a wired headset or speaker phone.

Steve: Bottom line time.

Karen: Bottom line, gentlemen. Smartphones are not going away. We rely on them every day for business calls, personal calls and viewing YouTube on the run ... oh yeah, for things like email, too. The way to minimize your radiation risk is to limit the amount of time your phone is next to your body, such as in your pocket or next to your ear.

Steve: If you want to see how much radiation your phone is putting out, compared to others, visit the Resources section of Karen's website at KarenRothNutrition.com and click on the Resources tab for Cell Phone Radiation. The Environmental Working Group (EWG) is a public-health watchdog group based in Washington DC, and they cut through the crap and will give you straightforward information you can trust.

Is Your Sunscreen Killing Your Manliness?

Steve: If you're one of the millions of Americans who use sunscreen, good for you … and bad for you depending on which brand you use. Like all consumer products, some are good for you while others are slowly kicking your butt down the alley, without you even knowing it.

Karen: If your sunscreen contains either oxybenzone, octinoxate, homosalate, parabens or octisalate, my suggestion is to just throw it away. These chemicals are supposed to help protect you from ultraviolet rays, but the first four are potential hormone disrupters. As an example, oxybenzone, the first on the list, can lower your testosterone, which means while you're out in the sun doing studly things at the beach, golf course, or on your bike, you may be losing your manlihood as this stuff soaks into your open, sweaty pores and goes to work on your system.

Steve: In animal studies, octinoxate showed disruption to thyroid and estrogen hormones. Oh, and the fifth one on the list, octisalate, is known to give some people red, sore or inflamed skin.

Karen: Now I'm not one to bring up problems without providing solutions, so here goes … As mentioned in the last section on cell phones, the Environmental Working Group (EWG) is a great resource for consumer information. They have an extensive database of over seven hundred name-brand sunscreens to help consumers like you fill in the information gap caused by the FDA's failure to set meaningful sunscreen standards.

Steve: I visited the site right after Karen saw which sunscreen I was using. Needless to say, I shot a three-pointer into our trash can with my sunscreen.

Karen: The EWG's sunscreen database lists products that offer the best combination of safety and effectiveness. It looks at the safest chemicals, the best sunburn protection, what prevents long-term sun damage that ages and wrinkles you, and what helps you prevent Cancer.

Steve: Check out your sunscreen on this list, and if yours was like mine, beat your woman to the three-pointer and slam dunk it!

Karen: You may be surprised to learn that 84% of the 785 sunscreen products analyzed by the EWG with an SPF rating of 15 or higher offer "inadequate" protection from the sun, or contain possibly unsafe ingredients.

Steve: I was amazed to learn that some popular sunscreen chemicals actually break down when exposed to sunlight. That's like having car wax that attracts bird crap. Okay, not the best analogy but you get my drift. Other brands simply soak in the skin and cause health concerns.

Karen: As mentioned in the prior section, you can visit my website, at KarenRothNutrition.com, and click on the Resources tab. There you'll find a link to the Environment Working Group's Sunscreen Guide.

Steve: Bottom line. There's no reason sunscreen shouldn't protect you while being safe for you. After all, isn't that the whole idea of protection?

Karen: You know, I have to say, you're getting much better at your bottom lines.

Steve: Thanks. I've been watching the way you do yours.

Karen: Thank you.

Steve: And I do the opposite.

Karen: Wouldn't want it any other way.

Steve: Really?

Karen: Just makes mine shine even more. Gotcha.

Steve: I hate when she does that.

For a boatload of healthy product suggestions, visit:
IMarriedaNutritionist.com
Click on "Karen's Selections."

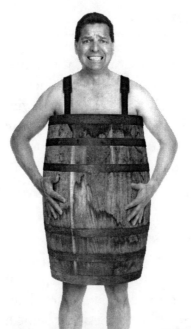

THE BODY STUFF

CHAPTER 7

*"To keep the body in good health is a duty ... otherwise we shall not be able to keep our mind strong and clear." ~ **Buddha***

*"If you don't keep your body in good health, you may have difficulty making a doody!" ~ **Steve Roth***

Allergies Blow – Here's How Not To

Steve: Allergies suck, there's just no way around it. In addition to making your nose run, eyes itch, and head feel like a balloon, they can really alter your quality of life and screw up some weekend play time.

Karen: A lot of people take antihistamines, which can provide some relief. However, they can cause side effects such as drowsiness, depression, and digestive upset.

Steve: You know, it wasn't until I was in my forties that a doctor actually explained that antihistamines can cause problems, as well as provide relief. He said that drying up your sinuses with antihistamines can also clog the tiny drainage hole at the bottom of the sinus cavity and cause sinus infections! Why didn't somebody tell me this before?

Karen: Seems some doctors have an "If you don't ask, I won't tell you" policy.

Steve: Afraid so. Okay, let's switch gears. I'm now going to share some "natural" remedies for allergies that Karen has shared with me. The first, and perhaps best thing that's ever worked for me, I stumbled upon by accident. As you may have read, I shoot competitive archery. A while back, I dove heavy into golf lessons along with a little tennis and I came down with Tendonitis.

Karen: And that's when I suggested he start taking MSM in powder form. It dissolves in water and helps with joint and tendon inflammation.

Steve: I thought I was telling this story.

Karen: You paused. I thought that meant I was to take over.

Steve: No pause, but that's okay. Go ahead.

Karen: No, it was a pause.

Steve: Actually, I was pondering.

Karen: Well, next time you decide to ponder, give me a signal.

Steve: Like what?

Karen: How about you put your index finger to your chin and stare into space.

Steve: That'll work.

Karen: MSM is an organic sulphur-containing nutrient, a naturally occurring compound in the environment and in the human body. It's needed for healthy skin, hair, nails, joints, and bones. As it turns out, MSM also prevents allergens from sticking to the respiratory tract, reducing allergy reaction.

Steve: After taking MSM for a few days, I suddenly noticed that I could sweep the patio and work in the backyard during heavy allergy season and have zero reaction. I even got out the blower and walked through a dust cloud on the patio. That I would not recommend, but I was in *Consumer Reports* Testing Mode so it just happened. That dust may have coated me from head to toe, but it did nothing to my allergies.

Karen: Tell them about the cats.

Steve: A friend of mine has four cats.

Karen: Five cats.

Steve: A few really big ones.

Karen: Not so big, just mainly furry.

Steve: Big ones. Anyway, every time I went over his house, bam. I would have a reaction. Sneezing. Watery eyes. When I started taking MSM, all that changed.

Karen: It was pretty amazing.

Steve: I can't vouch for the quality of the MSM on store shelves, but I can vouch for the MSM I use from Karen's website store. Not a plug, that's just the one I can vouch for. Up to you where you get it, but it might be worth investigating if you suffer from allergies.

Karen: Okay, let's shift gears and talk about quercetin and nettles.

Steve: A winning combination that is a great holistic product for allergies.

Karen: Quercetin is a bioflavonoid with powerful antihistamine and anti-inflammatory properties. Its antihistamine function can prevent the sneezing, itching, and swelling of an allergic reaction. Nettle leaf also has anti–inflammatory properties. And you're right, together they are an effective remedy for allergies.

Steve: Yes, I have friends who swear by the quercetin nettles combination for allergy relief, all year round.

Karen: Another good remedy is xylitol nasal spray, which helps wash away pollen and reduce allergy symptoms.

Steve: So there you have it, guys. Some good thoughts when it comes to allergy relief.

Karen: If you can get the job done naturally, it's the best way to go.

Steve: The bottom line on allergies, guys. There are some terrific and effective natural alternatives to eliminate the sneezing, wheezing, coughing, and blowing. Give 'em a try. It may be worth your while.

Length Matters!

Steve: There's a long-lived mistaken belief that the size of a man's nose, his feet, measurement of his wrist to index finger, and even his hand size reflects the size of his Johnson … and we're not talking outboard motors. I'm sure as much as women would love to have a reliable predictor for the expected height of the pup tent in their sheets the next morning, I'm sorry to say a reliable, scientific correlation just doesn't exist.

Karen: Pup tent?

Steve: You're right. That's too small. Let's go with circus tent.

Karen: Sometimes I think YOU belong in a circus tent.

Steve: Hey, I resemble that remark! Urologists at St. Mary's Hospital and University College Hospital in London put the foot myth to rest when they measured the length of 104 limp schlongs of men with various foot sizes. The predictions just didn't measure up. Some men with big feet were hung like mice, while others in the shoe size 8 zone were equipped with ginormous kick-stands.

Karen: Seriously? This is what we're spending research dollars on?

Steve: Wait, there's a method to my madness. Guys, you'll be happy to know that the average man is packing a whopping 3.5 inches of heat-seeking love missile. And when that beef bayonet is erect, the average guy's length is 5.1 inches … not the whopping 10 inches shown in porn movies or underwear ads. We'll now pause while you go get your ruler. Look, I know you want to so just go ahead and get it over with. Remember to close the blinds; it's not something the neighbors really want to see.

Karen: I really think we should get to the meat of the subject? I mean, oh, never mind.

Steve: Okay, guys. Now that we have the whole measuring thing out of the way, we need to discuss the length of your ring and index fingers, and how that measurement could affect your long-term health. I first read about this in *Men's Health* magazine and then in *Men's Journal* magazine, two of my favorite reads.

Karen: Oh, so now you're going to talk about health?

Steve: It's always been about health.

Karen: Right.

Steve: If your ring finger is longer than your index finger, what scientists call the digit ratio, you were more likely to have been exposed to excess testosterone in the womb. What that may translate into is a longer One Eyed Willy, higher IQ, a higher risk of prostate cancer and lower risk of heart attack. You may also be more physically aggressive than men with longer index fingers and you're probably mentally tough and optimistic, which is good if you're an air traffic controller and there's a plane coming in for landing up-side-down.

Karen: You're also more likely to have better athletic performance.

Steve: That, too. Take a look at these hands. What do you see?

Karen: Longer ring fingers. So that's why you're so good at archery, golf, bowling, tennis and petting the dog.

Steve: Exactly. By the way, I should note that this information comes out of a new study from the University of Florida.

Karen: Go Gators.

Steve: How'd you know that?

Karen: What?

Steve: Gators.

Karen: There are alligators in Florida.

Steve: Okay. Lucky reference.

Karen: Now, I also want to point out that if your index finger is longer than your ring finger, you were most likely exposed to less testosterone before birth which means you may be one-third less likely to develop Prostate Cancer. In addition, you may be half as likely to develop Osteoarthritis, and your sperm count may be on the low side.

Steve: You read the same articles, didn't you?

Karen: Of course.

Steve: You're tricky like that. Okay, bottom line, guys. When it comes to your length downstairs, it's skill over size. When it comes to length of your index and ring fingers, size may matter!

Vitamin D and Me

Steve: Okay, this is a huge health tip we're going to pass along. It's buried deep within this book for a reason. It's protected.

Karen: What? You think someone's going to steal it?

Steve: No. It's just that we guys are into protection.

Karen: Well, some are.

Steve: This health tip is probably one of the most important things I've learned from my nutritionist, and one of the most important things you'll probably read in this book. Okay, you're up to bat.

Karen: Many Americans falsely believe that they get a sufficient amount of vitamin D in milk, through their multivitamin, or they feel spending some time in the sunshine will do the trick. Well, the truth is unless you're a nudist and spend 30 minutes a day in direct sunshine or you're drinking truck-loads of milk each day …

Steve: Or you're naked and drinking truck-loads of milk, in the sunshine …

Karen: … Then you're most likely not getting enough vitamin D.

Steve: And that's a big problem, right? I know the answer; I'm just teeing it up.

Karen: Yes, it's a problem. It's estimated that somewhere around 90% of all Americans are deficient or have suboptimal levels of vitamin D. That deficiency puts people at risk for a host of very serious health conditions, including Autoimmune Disease, high blood pressure, prostate problems, Diabetes, Osteoporosis, Arthritis, Multiple Sclerosis, Heart Disease, among others.

Steve: Pretty serious stuff. Vitamin D also strengthens your immune system and helps you fight off infections, colds, and flu.

Karen: Vitamin D also improves cardiovascular health by easing calcification of your blood vessels.

Steve: And for all the guys who are working out, or not working out and wishing they were working out ... vitamin D strengthens muscles so you can work out at optimal efficiency. It also speeds up your metabolism.

Karen: Vitamin D also improves your mood.

Steve: Yes, it does improve your mood.

Karen: Why are you looking at me?

Steve: Nothing.

Karen: You're not suggesting ...

Steve: Certainly not.

Karen: Good. Vitamin D also strengthens your bones and teeth. It works better than fluoride for hardening teeth and preventing dental decay.

Steve: And now for the really big benefit of maintaining optimal levels of Vitamin D. New research now shows that the average person can reduce their risk of getting Cancer by 77% by simply ensuring their vitamin D levels are where they should be.

Karen: Makes you wonder why more attention hasn't been put on this simple approach to Cancer prevention.

Steve: Yeah, you would think health insurers would be all over this. Imagine how much they could slash their enormous payouts for Cancer treatments, chemotherapy, and hospital stays.

Karen: According to NaturalNews.com, 98% of conventional Cancer treatments not only fail miserably, but are also almost guaranteed to make Cancer patients sicker.

Steve: On the flip side to all of this, Cancer is a $200 billion industry for healthcare providers, hospitals, and especially big pharma. Wacky, I tell you.

Karen: Unfortunately, the mindset of our country has always been on dealing with problems when they occur, rather than preventing the problems from occurring in the first place.

Steve: Okay, so what level of vitamin D should the average person maintain for optimum health?

Karen: According to the Vitamin D Council ...

Steve: There's a Vitamin D Council? How do you get appointed to that? I'm guessing it's not having "Ds" on your report card.

Karen: I doubt that! Studies show that for proper health, your serum vitamin D levels should be a minimum of 50 ng/mL (125 nmol/L) with **optimal** levels falling between 50-80 ng/mL (125-200 nmol/L). These values apply to both children and adults.

Steve: And I suppose a lab test will confirm your current levels?

Karen: Absolutely. When you get a physical, make sure the doctor orders a vitamin D panel in your lab tests. Sometimes they resist, but that's when you insist!

Steve: Nice! Now, what about if your vitamin D levels are too high?

Karen: Vitamin D toxicity is extremely rare. In most cases, it can be corrected without lasting problems, provided that the body has not remained at that high level for too long. Too high a level of vitamin D, which can cause Hypercalcemia, can lead to soft tissue calcification, resulting in deposits of calcium crystals in the heart, lungs, and/or kidneys.

Steve: But wouldn't you say most people are deficient in vitamin D, rather than having too high a level.

Karen: Absolutely. About the only way your vitamin D levels will be too high is if you're supplementing with very high doses per day for an extended period of time.

Steve: Now, when it comes to buying vitamin D, what should people look for?

Karen: The important thing to remember is that not all vitamin D is the same, so make sure you do your research and find a reputable brand. You want to take vitamin D3, not D2.

Steve: It gives me huge peace of mind knowing that my vitamin D levels are right where they should be. It's like I have a security blanket against some really serious health conditions.

Karen: I couldn't agree more. Vitamin D is inexpensive and a game changer when it comes to your health.

Steve: Bottom line, guys. If you do nothing else from what you learned in this book, get your vitamin D level checked. This is a big one!

Sleep Is Nothing to Yawn About

Karen: Most people need 7-8 hours of sleep a night. But for over 60 million Americans who suffer with insomnia, it ain't happening.

Steve: Perhaps they're dealing with stress, or ultra-busy schedules or even Sleep Apnea, a disorder of having one or more pauses in breathing or shallow breaths during sleep. Regardless of the cause, we're a society that's sleep-deprived and it's making us sick.

Karen: Aside from being less alert and not thinking clearly, lack of sleep opens you up to all sorts of problems. For example, when you sleep, your body makes T-cells that help you fight colds and infection. If you don't get enough shut-eye, your internal army may be fighting without a platoon.

Steve: Nice military analogy!

Karen: I thought you would like that.

Steve: Indeed I did.

Karen: Lack of sleep also messes with your hormones and can cause you to actually gain weight.

Steve: A collective uh-oh!

Karen: To compound things, when you're tired, you're more likely to indulge in bad foods such as candy bars, chips, and fast food.

Steve: Sleep deprivation can also cause Microsleeps, a condition where the brain automatically shuts down, falling into a sleep state that can last from a second to a half minute. It's kinda like a mini-blackout where the person is not consciously aware its happening. Ever look at a sleepy person who appears to have checked out?

Karen: You. Last night while watching TV.

Steve: I was just deep in thought. I was also checking my eyelids for holes.

Karen: More like, checked out. Elvis had left the building. Microsleeps can also be very dangerous. Imagine driving down the highway at 65 miles per hour and not being present for 30 seconds.

Steve: Elvis has just crashed his car.

Karen: Assuming you don't have a medical condition that's preventing you from catching your zzzz's, here's four things that will help you get a better night's sleep. Number one. The body needs darkness to sleep. Light ramps up your wake cycle and counters your attempts to get a good night sleep. Make your bedroom as dark as possible.

Steve: If you need to turn on a light to find the john in the middle of the night, consider getting a seeing eye dog or practice the route blindfolded. Perhaps you can follow a string from the headboard to the toilet seat. Either way, avoid turning on a light whenever possible.

Karen: Number two. Cocktails, wine, and beer may relax you before bed, but they will fight with your sleep cycle. Alcohol fuels a neurotransmitter that, at first, makes you feel sleepy but look out. When the alcohol is metabolized, about 4 hours into your sleep cycle, and your liver's done with its filtering job, your brain kicks in gear and makes your sleep game's second half a challenging one.

Steve: I'll do number three. When you sleep, your body temperature drops. Yes, your partner can literally be giving you the cold shoulder. Sleeping in a cool room helps the temperature-drop process. A warm room only delays things.

Karen: And number four. Exercising is not only good for you, it helps you sleep better. But exercising too close to shut-eye time is not a good thing. Your body takes about 4-6 hours to cool down after exercising, and if that overlaps with your pillow time, you may have problems dozing off.

Steve: Bottom line, guys. Sleep is important. Get some.

Karen: Wow. That was amazingly to the point.

Steve: Yeah, well I'm in a hurry. It's time for my nap.

Breakfast of Skinny Champions

Steve: Karen shared with me a long time ago that you can drop weight and reduce fat by eating a high protein/healthy fat breakfast which kicks your fat-burning metabolism into high gear. On the flip side, a low-fat, high-carb breakfast increases appetite and causes you to hold on to fat.

Karen: You're a good study.

Steve: Well, when you're home schooled by a nutritionist, you absorb by default!

Karen: Yes, I guess you do.

Steve: Before I met Karen, my breakfasts used to be comprised of a lot of cereal and milk. These days my breakfasts often include hard boiled eggs, some cottage cheese, and avocado. I can't remember the last time I had cereal.

Karen: With the right breakfast, you can literally program your metabolism for the rest of the day.

Steve: Karen's home school program has taught me that eating a low-fat, high-carb breakfast causes your bad cholesterol to go up, along with your triglycerides and blood sugar. Regardless of how many calories you eat or how much exercise you get, it can set you up for Diabetes, Heart Disease, and Stroke.

Karen: Our ancestors thrived on foods like eggs, meat, and fish. This is what gave them power, strength, and vitality. Today, many people thrive on quick, convenient meals often heavy in carbs like bagels, toast, and cereal.

Steve: Eating a solid high protein/healthy fat breakfast will make you feel good all day with no mid-morning and mid-afternoon crash. You know, that 2:30 head nod where if you were at an auction, you could accidentally bid on a million dollar bottle of wine.

Karen: Some healthy-fat/protein breakfast items could include eggs; bacon, sausage, steak, and chicken from clean sources; avocado; and a whey protein smoothie made with coconut milk.

Steve: Karen's Muffin Eggs are amazing. They're a perfect heat-up option when you're in a hurry.

Karen: Bottom line, gentlemen. With a proper breakfast, you shouldn't be hungry, and cravings will seem to vanish. You'll notice it's easier to drop weight, and you'll feel like exercising again. Check out my Muffin Egg recipe on my website at KarenRothNutrition.com. They're packed with protein, easy to make, and really delicious!

Steve: Short, sweet, and to the point.

Karen: That's the best description of you I've heard in a long time.

Steve: Hey, I'm not that short. I'm 5'8 … on a good day.

Karen: What's a good day?

Steve: Any day I'm not 5'7½".

Karen: You're silly.

Steve: Yep, silly, sweet, and to the point. Silly replaces short. Here, I'll write that down for you.

Karen: Good. And while you have that pen out, draw a happy face on your forehead.

Steve: Why?

Karen: Because if you want to be silly, you may as well look silly!

Are Her Hormones Driving You Crazy?

Steve: Being married to a holistic nutritionist who specializes in hormone balancing, I've learned quite a bit about hormones and women. One important thing is that women who are dealing with hormonal issues can, at times, be a guy's worst nightmare.

Karen: You need to clarify that not all women experience hormonal issues the same.

Steve: Point well made. Guys, you may luck out if the woman in your life, who's dealing with hormonal issues, doesn't become your worst nightmare. Not all of them do but some have that ability.

Karen: Maybe it would help to explain what a woman with hormone imbalance is feeling.

Steve: Good point. Hormonal imbalance can put a woman on an emotional and physical roller-coaster that makes her feel like crap. It's just like how you feel when you're down and out, hung over, or stressed to the max. You don't want to deal with anyone, and if you do, it may not be pleasant.

Karen: You make some very good points in a weird guy sorta way.

Steve: Now, most guys are task oriented. When there's a problem, they immediately start looking for a solution. And the good news is, there are some real solutions for helping that special whacked out woman in your life who's dealing with hormonal issues.

Karen: I think "whacked out" is a bit extreme, don't you?

Steve: Okay, how about "hormonally challenged?"

Karen: Better.

Steve: So, guys, here's the playing field. A woman with hormonal issues has several options. One … do nothing and stick it out. This is old school and often how her mother, aunt, and women in black-and-white movies did it. Problem is the "sticking it out" phase can last years, and that means you're miserable, too ... by association.

Karen: Unfortunately, that is often the case.

Steve: Number two. A woman can take the pharmaceutical approach and start taking something called HRT which stands for hormone replacement therapy. Pop the drugs, perhaps feel better, but it greatly increases her risk for Cancer and other medical problems.

Karen: Absolutely.

Steve: Number three is something called bioidentical hormones.

Karen: The jury is still out on the possible long-term effects of putting these types of plant hormones in the human body. Several doctors and practitioners I respect are fine with bioidenticals as they may be beneficial to some women if closely monitored.

Steve: And finally, number four. In many cases, your wife can solve her hormone problems safely and naturally by allowing the body to rebalance itself. That's the way Karen approaches things with her clients. Rather than just dealing with the symptoms, you fix the root of the problem.

Karen: It's a bit more work, but I have helped hundreds of women across the country balance their hormones the natural way. It begins with a lab test to see where the hormone levels are. I then work with my clients to adjust their diets, add a few natural supplements, and oftentimes I suggest lifestyle changes. The result is, the body slides back into balance naturally. Sometimes it takes a few weeks, other times longer, but it's rolling with nature, not bucking it.

Steve: Okay, so why am I telling this to you guys? For one thing, most guys at some point are going to be on the receiving end of the effects of hormone imbalance, whether it comes from a wife, girlfriend, lover, mother, or woman undercover.

Karen: Nice rhyme.

Steve: Thank you. **Bottom line, guys, and this is the last bottom line of the book. If that special woman in your life is having issues, it's important for you, as her guy, to understand the problem, understand the options available for her, and give support that leads to wise choices and safe solutions. You've invested a lot of time and effort in your relationship, protect your investment and enjoy life's ride together as much as humanly possible.**

Karen: Very well done.

Steve: Thank you. It brought a tear to my eye.

Karen: I'm glad you wanted to add this hormone section to the book.

Steve: Well, the truth is, I'm living with a hormone-balancing specialist. It only made sense to share some insights I've learned with the guys.

Karen: Indeed.

For a boatload of healthy product suggestions, visit:
IMarriedaNutritionist.com
Click on "Karen's Selections."

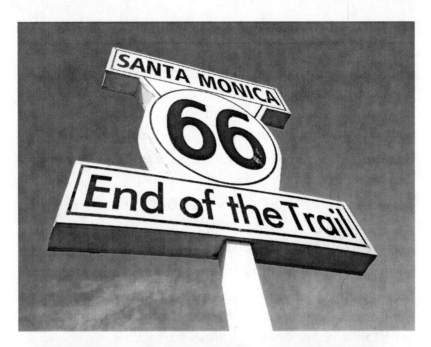

EPILOGUE STUFF

YOU HAVE TO END SOMEWHERE

Steve: Well, here we are at the end of the book.

Karen: Yes, and it's been fun.

Steve: It sure has. And, guys, what I'm most excited about is that we were able to share all this great inside information on health and nutrition. That was really cool. I'm hoping there were a few "Ah-Ha!" moments along the way.

Karen: Absolutely. And if you gentlemen make even a few small changes in your diet and lifestyle based on what you learned, you'll be that much healthier for it.

Steve: The reality is that you can live a long, healthy life if you take care of your body, rather than depending on medications to try to do it for you. As you grow old, don't just assume you're destined to be on all those drugs. Yes, some medications are necessary in certain circumstances, but you don't have to be a slave to the pharmaceutical industry. Empower yourself by taking control of your health. Ask questions.

Karen: Did you know that roughly 25% of all TV commercials airing in the US are for pharmaceuticals?

Steve: Actually, I didn't know that but I'm not surprised.

Karen: It was biochemist Linus Pauling, one of the most important scientists of the 20th century who said, "Optimum nutrition is the medicine of tomorrow." I couldn't agree more.

Steve: Pauling was right, and he had forty-eight honorary PhD degrees and two Nobel Prizes to back him up. If you nourish the body, it can oftentimes fix itself.

Karen: But here's the problem. Less than 6% of graduating physicians in the US receive any formal training in nutrition. It's no wonder doctors lean so heavily on pharmaceuticals; it's what they've been taught.

Steve: Pretty sad. Guys, I have one more point to make before we wrap this up. And it's a biggie. Staying healthy can help keep you out of the hospital.

Karen: And a hospital is not where you want to be unless it's absolutely necessary.

Steve: Karen and I recently watched a terrific documentary called *Food Matters*. It highlighted the fact that 80,000 people a year die in hospitals from infections and another 106,000 die due to adverse drug reactions. Yes, hospitals have their place in the world; just try not to make it a favorite destination. Besides, the food sucks.

Karen: Well, I guess that about does it for me.

Steve: Thanks so much for being my partner in crime with this book.

Karen: My pleasure. Every bad cop needs a good cop.

Steve: Right … I think.

Karen: I have to go feed Riley.

Steve: I can take it from here.

Karen: Gentlemen, it's been a pleasure. Take care and stay healthy. We need more healthy role models out there.

Steve: And with that … Karen Roth, MS, CNC has left the building! I mean, room. So, here we are again, just us guys. I guess this would be a good time to share a few parting thoughts. When I met Karen, I was like many of you trying my best to stay healthy. The problem is that there's so much conflicting information out there about what's good for you, what's not good for you, and it was all so confusing. Had I not married a nutritionist, I'm guessing I would probably be on Statins by now. I remember a doctor once mentioning something about my cholesterol being a little high. Plus, my dad was on Statins so it was predetermined, right? And I'm guessing I would probably be 25 pounds heavier than I am now because my dad was heavy and everyone knows that runs in the family, right? Actually, that's a weak excuse. Poor eating runs in families. But I did marry a nutritionist and that's when I began to sort out the truths versus the non-truths. Half of being healthy is having correct information; the other half is not being lazy and making some real changes in your life.

Each year when I get a physical, the doctor is always amazed by my lab results. Everything's where it should be and I'm able to deny the doctor his chance to give me a handful of pharmaceutical samples that his pharmaceutical rep gave him and the pharmaceutical company gave to her to give to him to give to me. It's a good feeling to be in control. The path isn't always easy, but the results are so satisfying.

Lastly, when I turned fifty, I visualized that I was stepping onto the first tee box of the back-9. I remember looking back on a lot of adventures that happened on the front-9, most of them good, others challenging, and yet others chalked up as learning experiences. Yes, I remember thinking where I am today is where I'm happy to be. When you reach the mid-point in your life, you have a different perspective of the world around you. For me, the bird's eye view of this whole crazy world of ours actually started to make sense, like connecting the dots. And now, as I look forward, I see a lot of fairway ahead of me. I made a commitment to myself long ago that I'll do whatever it takes to make that final 18th hole putt standing erect (without Viagra), showing off my real teeth as I smile and wave to the crowd, and looking back over the entire course without regrets knowing I took the time to learn the game, make informed decisions, and played it well. What could be more satisfying?

That's all for now. Cheers, guys, and we'll see you out on the course.

Steve

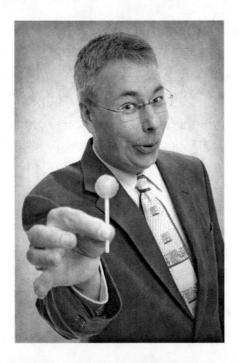

ACKNOWLEDGEMENT STUFF

THE THANKING BEGINS

Thank you. Thank you. Thank you. And thank you, again!

We wish to thank everyone who helped us along our journey to getting this book written and published. Most importantly, we wish to thank:

Robin Quinn, our devoted editor, for helping us dot our I's, cross our T's, and for the overall guidance she provided from beginning to end.

James Arneson, our book cover designer and formatter who pulled out all the stops so we can honestly say that you can judge a book by its cover!

Steven Bridges, our outstanding photographer who helped us capture just the right moment for our book cover. He also shot the photo on our "About the Authors" page!

David Nichols and **Nutritionist Diane Reich** who proofread our book and provided some amazing feedback.

Dr. Joseph Collins, Harry Thomason, Tony Scott, Damon Goddard, Todd Greene, and **David Nichols** for taking time out of their busy schedules to share their opinions about our book in quotes for the back cover.

Tyler Roth, Steve's grown son, who has proven you can adopt a healthy diet at a young age, live a healthy lifestyle through college, be all muscle with a six-pack, climb the highest peaks, board the steepest slopes, and be able to enjoy life to its fullest if you stay healthy.

And finally …

Riley, our beagle, for letting us end the book with a picture of his back-side.

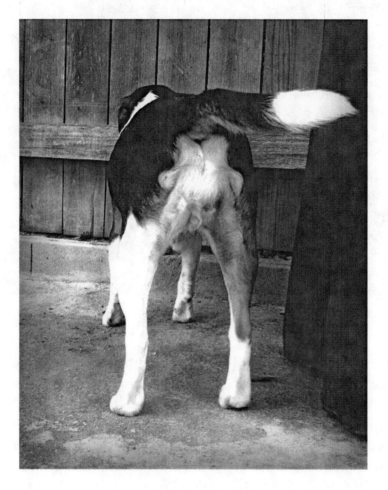

THE END.

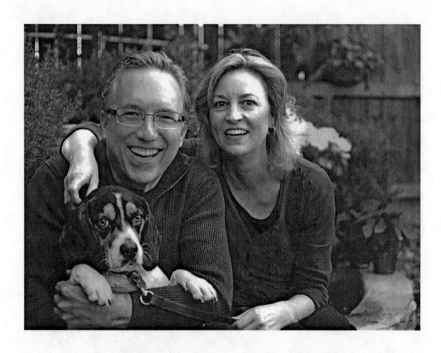

ABOUT THE AUTHORS

Steve Roth spent a good part of his career working all around the entertainment business. As a television comedy writer, he worked on a variety of network, cable, and syndicated TV programs, from the CBS hit series *Designing Women* to Nickelodeon's first live-action series, *Hey Dude*. In addition to TV, Steve produced, directed, and wrote the experimental feature film comedy *Vacation Survivors* which premiered in Los Angeles and screened at the Independent Feature Film Market in New York City and at the Santa Clarita Film Festival. Outside of entertainment, Steve has worked for a number of years in the area of advertising and marketing. In the athletic arena, Steve is a competitive archer who can hit a tea cup at 60 yards, an average golfer who tries to keep it in the fairway, and a dedicated exerciser who works out in his home gym.

Karen Roth, MS, CNC holds a Master of Science Degree in Holistic Nutrition from Hawthorn University and earned her undergraduate degree from University of California, Irvine. Karen has been featured on national television, in print publications such as *USA Today,* has served as a radio host, and is an active social media blogger and public speaker. As a holistic nutritionist, Karen shares her knowledge to empower her clients and others to take control of their health with food choices that best support their specific health condition. A specialist in hormone balancing, Karen believes that every ill health condition can benefit and possibly improve from a solid foundation of healthy food choices.

Karen and Steve reside in the Los Angeles area with their beagle, Riley who loves to snack on fresh organic vegetables.

CPSIA information can be obtained at www.ICGtesting.com
Printed in the USA
LVOW132133130313

324193LV00003B/154/P